Drug Addiction and Drug Policy

Drug Addiction and Drug Policy

The Struggle to Control Dependence

Edited by
Philip B. Heymann
William N. Brownsberger

Harvard University Press

Cambridge, Massachusetts
London, England / 2001

Library of Congress Cataloging-in-Publication Data

Drug addiction and drug policy: the struggle to control dependence/edited by Philip B. Heymann and William N. Brownsberger.
    p. cm.
Includes bibliographical references.
ISBN 0-674-00327-6 (alk. paper)
  1. Substance abuse–United States. 2. Substance abuse–United States–Prevention.
3. Drug abuse–United States–Prevention. 4. Drug abuse–Government policy–United States. 5. Narcotics, Control of–United States. 6. Drugs of abuse–Law and legislation–United States. I. Heymann, Phillip B. II. Brownsberger, William N.
RC564.65 .D785 2001
362.29′0973–dc21   00-054486

To Jim Harpel, whose belief in the project, enthusiasm, determination, good humor, and financial support made this book possible, with the appreciation of all the authors

Contents

Drug Addiction and Drug Policy

Introduction: Drug Policy with a New Focus

Philip B. Heymann

Policy analysts, doctors, and social scientists share a desire to be objective about facts, clear and logical in their choice of concepts, and rigorous in their recommendations. They do not want to be seen as carrying values, with which others might readily disagree, into their arguments—obscuring the facts, distorting clear thought, or using emotion to persuade.

In one important sense, the authors of the chapters in this book fit within this mold. They are social scientists, medical doctors, and policy analysts. They are eager to add new factual knowledge to the bewildering array of considerations that affect the choice of drug policy, whether it be knowledge about the demographics of drug dependence and sales or about the conditions of self-control of a drug-dependent person. They wish to clarify concepts, from the possible forms of prevention to the seemingly arbitrary limitation that prevents our using social policy to further drug policy and vice versa. They are rigorous in their forms of persuasion, whether that involves recognizing that drug use is a "multi-attribute" problem or building testing into an ingenious proposal for "mandatory abstinence."

But at a deeper level, there is another dimension to almost all these chapters. Without ignoring familiar ways of seeking objectivity, each of the authors is wrestling with ethical issues that long preceded our modern faith in science, let alone the far more recent birth of policy analysis. The ancient Greeks were already worrying about whether there were times when we couldn't trust ourselves to act responsibly,

1

the ethics of paternalistic manipulation and coercion on behalf of another's well-being or character, the implications of political choices made for others whose values might differ, and how far defense of oneself and the values one hopes to transmit can justify harm to others. These questions have been turned, examined, and readdressed over many centuries. They reappear now.

New Understandings Affecting Drug Policy

There is a received model of drug policy. The familiar model begins by dividing the possible ways of dealing with harmful mind-altering drugs into three categories: prevention, treatment, and law enforcement. The model recognizes, although it often pays too little attention to, the fact that different drugs may demand different mixes of these three categories, either because one drug is more susceptible than others to particular ways of handling (only heroin can be treated with methadone) or because the harms of one drug are much less or much more than those of another.

Within each broad category there are a variety of programs—different forms of treatment, different forms of prevention, different forms and targets of law enforcement. For each of the subcategories, attempts have been made to evaluate its prospects and costs with different drugs in various situations. Ideally, this would permit a comparison of cost effectiveness within any category and even a comparison of best alternatives across the broad categories of law enforcement, treatment, and prevention.

Major problems of organization and politics further complicate policy choice in the United States. Organizationally, there is a division of responsibility for the various devices to control drug use among federal, state, and local governments and among an unusually large number of organizations at each level of government (including at the federal level those dealing with health, education, border control, national security, and criminal justice).

Whoever is in charge (a subject of constant contention) and whatever the goals that might be adopted by evaluators of drug policy (there is no agreement here) and whatever the evidence on the cost and effectiveness of various paths to those goals (too little is known here), choice of policy in the area of drugs is also a highly political matter. Presidents shudder when the percentage of high school students using marijuana goes up; they boast when the National Household Survey on Drug Abuse figures go down. So prevention programs, even ones that have shown no likelihood of success, are popular, although not as popular as heavy penalties for those who might introduce our children to drugs. Treatment programs are never a favorite: although addicts cause much harm, the harms from their behavior are not widely dispersed, collecting tightly around their families and neighborhoods and diminished by the addict having income or wealth; and addicts inspire very little public sympathy.

Like any model, this established one spotlights certain issues and obscures others in the shadows. The contributors to this book pull issues out of those shadows. Since there is reason to question how much more we can accomplish using the familiar model, exploring new ways of looking at the drug problem is extremely important. That is the aim of this book.

The chapters that follow begin by clarifying concepts and adding a new demographic dimension to the description of effects of drug policy. They go on to explore the implications of scientific knowledge about drug dependence. Then two authors analyze the implications of the remarkable overlap between the addicts who provide the greater part of the market for illegal drugs and the population arrested in any given year. Finally, two authors draw attention to a major approach to drug policy we have never taken, namely linking it to social policy.

New Conceptual and Demographic Maps

Two chapters present fresh overviews of the American drug problem. The first, by Mark H. Moore, provides a comprehensive and systematic set of categories in which to think about what causes and what reduces drug use and harms and thus about the fields in which various policy options can work. A convincing picture can be produced, Moore shows, out of the following pieces:

- Notions of individual propensities to use drugs and of their causes.
- A pattern describing the mix of propensities of a group of people in whom we are interested.
- A distribution of different patterns of actual use by different users reflecting both differences in dependence and the frequency of particularly harmful contexts of use.
- The available supply of drugs and the conditions that encourage or discourage that supply.
- Particular harms and adverse consequences from particular distributions of patterns of use, such as the risks that come with a pattern of using dirty needles to administer a drug.

Social and cultural factors shape propensities to use drugs and patterns of their use; they also affect the likely consequences of use in those patterns. Governmental policies, in turn, help shape these environmental factors. They also affect the conditions that make drugs more or less available to particular individuals at any particular time.

Moore's conceptual map provides a skeleton for thinking about drug policy. William N. Brownsberger's piece on drug users and drug dealers uses the available demographic information to add flesh and muscle to the skeleton. The existing measurement systems have grave weaknesses. The two major systems that measure prevalence, the Monitoring the Future survey of high school students and the broader National Household Survey on Drug Abuse, suffer from several serious limitations. Both rely on self-reports which lead to substantial underestimates. Both fail to interview those who have dropped out of school and households, a small fraction of the total population but rich in people with serious drug problems. Neither is a particularly effective way to study dependence or the population in need of treatment.

The other systems we use, measuring drug use by arrestees and emergency room admissions, are obviously not representative. So Brownsberger had to undertake original research to determine who is dealing drugs and/or dependent on drugs. He concludes that both dependence and dealing are found disproportionately in poverty areas and, perhaps, as a result, disproportionately among minority groups.

The obvious implication is that both criminal justice policies and the most harmful effects of drug use will have their greatest impacts in the same neighborhoods and among minority populations suffering from other disadvantages, even though drug users, as opposed to exceptionally heavy users, are probably spread fairly evenly throughout the population. As Jonathan P. Caulkins and Philip Heymann point out in a later chapter, the concentration in minority populations contributes importantly to the facts that as many as 30 percent of black youths are in some way under the control of the criminal justice system and that our prison populations have ballooned to many times what they were only a few years ago, largely with minority inmates.

Brownsberger also describes trends of use over time and their relationship to social attitudes toward particular drugs and perceptions of the dangerousness of those drugs. Two critical facts are hardly surprising: heavy cocaine or heroin use tends to result in high rates of criminal offending, and heavy users of cocaine or heroin are arrested quite frequently. The first is a natural consequence of the inability of many heavy users to hold well-paid positions and their resulting recourse to crime to pay the cost of drugs, a cost that is kept high by law enforcement. The second is an inevitable result of frequent offending. The combination creates interesting policy possibilities that are described later in the book by Mark A. R. Kleiman.

New Understandings of Dependence or Addiction and of Treatment

The chapters by Gene M. Heyman, Sally L. Satel, and George E. Vaillant take us from the macro-vision provided by conceptual maps and demography into the equally important, but far more sharply focused, issues concerning the meaning of dependence. What had been a familiar question addressed in terms of official specification of symptomatology suddenly took on new meanings with the entrance of neurobiology into the area. The new ability to see changes in the brain that accompany use and dependence brought with it suggestions that addiction was as beyond alteration by free will as a viral infection. These three chapters all aim at reasserting the primacy of human choice as a way of understanding and dealing with drug dependence, while recognizing but not surrendering to the rival claims some make on the basis of neurobiology.

New understandings of the circuitry in the brain that provides rewards and motivation and new techniques for observing the effect of drugs on the brain of a user or addict have provided a major challenge to what has been learned from observation of the behavior of addicted, dependent users. C. P. Snow wrote of the battle within universities between science and humanities. That battle is reproducing itself in discussions about the meaning of dependence. Neurobiologists can see and explain how almost all of the familiar drugs of abuse operate by redirecting the controls which release or restrain the neurotransmitters which provide motivation and reward.

The effects of heroin and cocaine on the brain can be observed in ways that the effects of ice cream or steak cannot. This suggests to the brain scientists a variety of policy possibilities. Perhaps antagonists could be developed that would prevent the effects of the illicit drugs. Perhaps we could learn to understand what drugs are substitutes for others by observing similar reactions within the brain. Perhaps in exploring the effects on the two critical neurotransmitters, dopamine and serotonin, we could also learn something more about the "gateway" effects of use of one drug on the use of another. Broadest of all would be the political effects: perhaps the public could be made to see addiction as a disease rather than as a moral failing.

Gene Heyman and Sally Satel argue in their chapters that making this view of addiction one's exclusive orientation is distorting and harmful. They point out the extensive evidence that addictive behavior can be altered by a recognition of adverse consequences from that behavior or by rewards for abstention. They recognize that dependence means compulsive use of a substance in face of harmful consequences, but they argue that consequences which are immediate and certain exercise an important influence over the continued use of a drug. The evidence they present ranges from experiments done on alcoholics to the natural experiment that occurred when large numbers of heroin-dependent soldiers returned from Vietnam.

The message for Satel is that getting over addiction requires extraordinarily hard work by the addict, in part because there are neurological changes that must be overcome. She urges the imposition of conditions in a variety of forms, including the use of criminal sanctions to require treatment. Coerced treatment, she points out, has better results than voluntary treatment partly because the results of any form of treatment depend upon its duration. She also recognizes what Gene Heyman emphasizes, that the individual needs alternative activities and greater prospects.

Both Satel and Heyman are skeptical of any cure that depends upon the regular use of a substitute drug or of an antagonist. Satel accepts the usefulness of methadone for heroin addicts but contrasts it with the equally good results that can be accomplished by residential treatment. Her message is that it is a human being, the addict himself, who must assume much of the responsibility for freeing himself from dependence on a drug, and that confusing the human being with a set of neurological pathways—substituting science for humanity—is a serious mistake.

Heyman's viewpoint is similar. It is he who gives us the complete account of the critical evidence. His recommendations emphasize the centrality of dealing with the life situation of an addict. He emphasizes the ability of contingencies to affect drug use, and the extent to which natural contingencies, coming about as part of the results of drug dependence, are likely to reinforce continued dependence. He addresses the question: Why is addiction so hard to end either alone or with treatment? The answer, he argues, is in part biological with the alteration of brain circuits but can as readily be thought of as the result of psychological laws of reward and punishment operating in the very peculiar context of great, immediate rewards, delayed punishments, and progressively narrowed options. Treatment fails so often, Heyman argues, because those who go into treatment are disproportionately those who have other psychological problems and diseases. Individuals with only a drug dependence to deal with have a much greater prospect of successful recovery.

There are no longitudinal studies that begin with a cohort of individuals representative of the population at large and follow them to discover the characteristics of those who come to use illicit drugs, those who become dependent on a particular drug, those who recover, those who return to use, and so on. But George Vaillant has developed such information with regard to those dependent on an addictive legal drug—alcohol.

Vaillant shares with Satel and Heyman a belief that addiction is voluntary behavior in the limited sense that it is subject to change when the addict is confronted with an environment changed in a variety of ways. Like Heyman, Vaillant believes in the importance of adding alternative, attractive structures to replace drugs in the life of the addict. He also believes in the importance of providing immediate and certain adverse consequences for relapse. But he makes the moral as well as the practical case for a particular pattern of treatment, which can take the form of conditions of parole or methadone maintenance or 12-Step processes or other procedures. Vaillant argues, in short, that a particular type of paternalism, with both its caring and its coercive aspects, is critical. And that form of paternalism must be the choice of the addict, even if it is a choice that is made because of adverse consequences threatened by employers or law enforcement. After choice comes structure and an array of carrots and sticks.

In the broadest way, Heyman, Satel, and Vaillant are all calling for a recognition that an addict is a human being behaving in an irresponsible way, perhaps as a result of severe social problems and limited opportunities, but needing to come to terms with his life. Seeing himself as the victim of brain disease will not help establish the conditions of self-determination and responsibility that are required for the extremely difficult task of recovery. Vaillant states the conditions of recovery that Satel and Heyman also endorse. They require demands on the individual coupled with concern. All agree that these can be brought about in a coercive form with as great effect as voluntarily. Each sees the cup of an addict's self-control as half full, not merely half empty. The task of treatment is not primarily to find a drug that will eliminate enough temptations to allow the individual to function with greatly reduced self-control. The task is to help him build self-control until he can handle the temptation of further use.

Implications for Dealing with Dependent Users

The distinctions among prevention, treatment, and law enforcement as ways of dealing with the problems of addiction are at least as misleading as they are helpful. As Moore argues, the social and moral effects (as well as the increased costs attributable to the deterrent effects) of law enforcement against users of, and dealers in, illegal drugs are a powerful form of prevention of use. The threat of criminal sanctions is just as effective as school-based prevention programs—which have been shown to affect not only attitudes and knowledge about drugs but also use of cigarettes and marijuana, with the effects of good junior high school interventions persisting at least into the twelfth grade. Similarly, law enforcement is a source of motivation to enter treatment. The risk of punishment for crimes of drug use or dealing and for crimes committed to pay for drug use and the inconvenience forced on dependent users by the threat of law enforcement can, and undoubtedly do, drive users toward treatment. But the connection can be even more specific.

The Department of Justice tests arrestees in a number of jurisdictions for evidence of recent drug use. The figures are remarkably high. The converse is also true. A very high percentage of frequent users of illicit drugs (other than marijuana)—Mark Kleiman estimates three-quarters for cocaine—are arrested in the course of a year. Combining this information with the evidence that Satel sets forth that coerced treatment is at least as effective as voluntary treatment and, in absolute terms, has very good results adds up to an invitation to build a new set of policies to reduce the size of the drug markets, reduce the number of crimes committed by heavy users, and improve addicts' lives. The new policies would consciously use law enforcement to coerce treatment or, more directly, abstention from use.

There are two familiar ways of forcing treatment on a drug user by law enforcement. The first delays prosecution if the defendant will go into treatment and forgoes prosecution if the defendant stays in treatment. The second puts a judge in charge of meeting regularly with defendants who have been referred to a drug court. The judge is responsible for encouragement and sanctions designed to keep the defendant off drugs. Both programs are generally available only to people who have not committed serious or repeated offenses, but even so they can impose a substantial burden on limited treatment facilities.

Kleiman argues for an alternative that is cheaper and that could be applied to a far broader category of defendants. He proposes making probation or parole (after even a defendant whose crime is serious has served some part of the sentence for that crime) conditional on regular drug testing. A defendant who failed a drug test would be subject to an absolutely certain but relatively mild penalty. Treatment would be reserved for those who seemed unable to comply even with sanctions that were sure and swift. This regimen would be applied systematically to any offender who tested positive for illicit drugs on arrest. Preliminary evaluations of an experimental program in the District of Columbia suggest that the proposal has real promise. Kleiman argues that it could greatly reduce the size of the market for illicit drugs, the number of crimes committed by drug-using offenders, and the amount of damage to family and associates caused by offenders.

Kleiman's idea is bold and plausible, and, at the high end of reasonable hopes, promises very dramatic benefits. Its payoff could be immense, depending upon what fraction of heavy drug users can be deterred by a scheme of short but certain sanctions. The arguments of Satel and Heyman suggest that the fraction may be large. But the proposal has one obvious weakness. It imposes difficult tasks on criminal justice networks and places the major responsibility for these on already overburdened, often failing probation departments.

William N. Brownsberger, in his chapter on this same proposal, questions whether the payoff from a program of coerced abstinence is likely to be as large as Kleiman suggests. For many relatively light users of drugs, the crime rates are not particularly high and are not likely to be affected by a successful program of ending drug use. For highly dependent users, Brownsberger argues, the short sanctions proposed by Kleiman are not likely to work. Nor is it important to use drug testing to determine their heavy dependence and thus the likelihood of their resort to crime to pay for the habit. Other detection devices will often work as well. In particular, Brownsberger believes, the addicted offender needs treatment of the sort described by Heyman, Satel, and Vaillant. Coerced abstinence may help during the period of probation and parole but not thereafter. That leaves, as the only population likely to be responsive to coerced abstinence, those who are in the middle ranks of drug users in terms of their use and the amount of crime they commit to support that use. The maximum payoff of the program depends upon the size of that group.

In only one situation, but an important one, Brownsberger favors Kleiman's proposal without reservation. In the world of drug control, the most dangerous situation may be an epidemic in which an initial enthusiasm for a new drug spreads rapidly through the population well before the adverse consequences become obvious. The model is the cocaine epidemic that began in the 1980s. As Jonathan Caulkins has argued elsewhere, it is very difficult to imagine a prevention program (one that relies on schools, television, or other forms of education directed at drug use) that could be put in place quickly enough to be of any use at a time of epidemic. Brownsberger notes that at such a time coerced abstinence may be particularly useful to eliminate the contagious effect of seeing one's friends using a new and apparently attractive drug before its high costs in health, education, work, and so on become apparent. In sum, he regards Kleiman's proposal as potentially useful on a selective basis, but not on the automatic and universal basis urged by Kleiman. The difference in views powerfully suggests the desirability of experiments with such programs.

Two Further Implications

The arguments of those in favor of legalizing or decriminalizing the distribution or use of some or all drugs that are now illegal focus on the costs that are generated by law enforcement as an instrument of drug policy. The costs are real, although most people believe that the costs of a policy of "legalization"—costs that would flow from the predictable increase in drug use and dependence—would be far greater, at least for most drugs and for very large segments of the American population. But holding such a belief and being opposed to abandoning law enforcement does not make it reasonable to fail to tailor law enforcement in a way to reduce social costs and it does not make it sensible to fail to take preventive steps of social policy which might reduce the demand for the drug and, therefore, the amount of law enforcement required to deal with that demand. Nor does it mean that we should fail to use other social programs to compensate those who disproportionately bear the costs of drug enforcement. In different ways, these are the issues addressed by Jonathan P. Caulkins and Philip Heymann and then by David Boyum and Peter Reuter.

Caulkins and Heymann address the problem of massive, readily replaceable numbers of lower-level street dealers, who for more than a decade have been incarcerated for much longer periods in much larger numbers. The authors reject legalization and, therefore, recognize that a black market will persist. They see little reason to question the wisdom of long sentences for drug kingpins. But they question the sentences given to street dealers. Justice requires punishment for selling drugs, but not punishment as severe and as arbitrarily distributed as it is now. Social policy requires keeping the price of drugs high and the availability limited, but not ignoring the immense costs associated with mandatory extended prison terms for many of the hundreds of thousands of individuals selling illicit drugs in very small transactions. The marginal benefits of locking up high percentages of low-level dealers seem small indeed.

Caulkins and Heymann believe that the present structure of sentencing by most states and the federal government involves two forms of mistake. First, the costs and benefits of various sentencing options are addressed separately from the many related questions of expenditures on arrest, prosecution, bail, and community supervision. For example, it is likely that investments at the earliest stages of drug law enforcement (increasing the chance of arrest) would be more effective in reducing drug use than longer sentences; that is strongly suggested by the successful efforts of New York and Boston in dealing with violence. Highly developed forms of community supervision under terms of probation or parole have equally dramatic prospects, especially in the light of modern technology.

The second mistake is just as important: decisions made by statute at a state or federal level necessarily ignore not only many relevant differences among individuals—which can be recognized by judges or prosecutors although at the cost of risking unequal treatment and confused deterrent messages—but also differences in the needs and concerns of different communities at different times. The latter differences can be considered in systems that don't risk unequal treatment and that maintain a clear deterrent message.

What is needed, Caulkins and Heymann argue, is a system that operates under consistent guidelines which incorporate the views of local communities, not just the views of larger jurisdictions, as to appropriate punishment. And such a system should encourage comparison of the benefits of expenditures on longer sentences with the benefits of resources spent at other stages of law enforcement such as policing or parole. The authors describe how one such system might work to recognize community values and community situations without sacrificing much of the goals of predictability and uniformity which led to the passage of state and federal mandatory minimum and guideline sentences.

Massive efforts at law enforcement, particularly addressed to retail dealing, have revealed sharp limits to our capacity to discourage use by denying access or raising still further the price of illicit drugs (which we have already made orders of magnitude higher than they would be if legal). We are well aware of the possibility that health care can help address problems of drug dependence. We also know that the relationships between law enforcement and medical treatment, on the one hand, and drug use and dependence, on the other, are complicated and sometimes flow in unanticipated directions or have unwanted consequences. To some extent, we have tried to deal with these complications. Surprisingly, Boyum and Reuter point out in the final chapter, there is far less exploration of the relationships between other aspects of social policy and drug use, abuse, or dependence. Could we, by opening this very wide avenue of exploration and potential experimentation, broadly supplement Kleiman's "regulatory" proposal for drug addicts and reduce the costs of our current emphasis on imprisoning low-level dealers? This is the central question for Boyum and Reuter.

They make a powerful case that drug use and drug law enforcement affect housing, health, education, employment, and so on. Less certainly, they argue, inadequacy of access to these benefits for the poor affects the amount of drug use. They then ask why we don't give greater consideration to these consequences as we design social policy or drug policy: that is, why these types of policies are not more accommodating and better neighbors to each other. The answer they furnish is a recommendation of caution for a wide-ranging set of reasons. Tracing the relations between these "neighbors" may be too hard and too uncertain. The distinctions made in trying to accomplish drug policy by manipulating social policy may be morally indefensible. The social programs that would have to be retargeted in some way may be too hidden in the various categories of the budgets of different agencies.

In the final analysis, it is hard to imagine each of the many purposes of a modern federal or state government being reflected in the activities of every separate agency of that government. Boyum and Reuter see little reason for broadly departing from the convenient pattern that encourages each agency to focus on only a few objectives. They doubt whether incorporating the reduction in drug use among the purposes of a number of additional social agencies would be productive, even if it were in all cases well motivated, and they doubt that it would always be well motivated.

Ethical Dimensions

One ethical issue has always divided people concerned about drug policy. No form of objective analysis could bridge most of the gap between those who believe deeply that giving up one's capacity for self-control—whether by intoxication or drug dependence—is immoral and, if tolerated, socially destructive and those who believe that the decision to abandon some measure of self-control is up to the individual, so long as he or she does not harm others. The difference carries over to attitudes toward addicts. Those in the latter group are more likely to treat addicts as in need of help; those in the former group, as deserving of the consequences of their immoral choices. But less obvious ethical issues also have very important effects on drug policy, as the authors discover and reveal.

Heyman, Satel, and Vaillant are plainly wrestling with the issue of how social institutions, public or private, should treat someone with diminished responsibility. They reject the "liberal" stance that addiction is a disease like any other, for which the individual cannot be held responsible. For them, treatment involves creating the conditions under which an individual can develop self-control. And one of those conditions, perhaps the most important, is an insistence that the person is responsible for what he does. On the other hand, they plainly do not believe that the addict deserves the benefits of the Kantian injunction that every person should always be treated as an end in himself and never as a means. They believe that certain forms of coercion and manipulation are necessary not only to the addict's welfare but also to his entitlement to be treated with the full dignity of a responsible individual.

They are exploring a new form of ethical judgement: the right to demand that someone lacking in self-control generate some measure of that self-control by determination, but to make this demand only when it is accompanied by the creation of coercive conditions that will support the individual's effort and that can be maintained by the individual when treatment is over.

Strangely closely related is an ethical issue that lies behind the chapter by Boyum and Reuter. Are there situations in which we cannot trust ourselves to act responsibly? If there are, what should we do then? In expressing doubts about the wisdom of linking our decisions on matters of social policy to their effects, sometimes substantial, on the use or sale of drugs, Boyum and Reuter are plainly troubled by the fear that we will not act responsibly, that the moral passion for attacking the sale and use of drugs will override all moral concern for the welfare of citizens who have failed to behave responsibly in using drugs.

The authors recognize the immense bureaucratic, legislative, and conceptual complexity of taking account of the effects of drug policy on the vast field of social policy and the effects of the latter on drug policy. But there is plainly more than this behind their reticence; there is a fear that the retributive and paternalistic urges that are released as we deal with drug policy may not be adequately contained as they spread into other areas. Like Odysseus resisting the sirens, we may have to bind ourselves if we are to refrain from actions that will have major effects on those who elicit more anger than concern.

Brownsberger, Caulkins, and Heymann address the issues of political choice that appear only after one has wrestled with these issues of paternalism. An economist looking at a choice of two regulatory schemes would be likely to focus on the issue of efficiency: which produces the greater total benefits for all the parties affected. References to the distribution of costs and benefits would often be casual or missing. The same is often true of discussions of drug policy. But how does all this really work out? Caulkins and Heymann display the extreme difficulty of speaking in terms of efficiency about the varied benefits and costs of even a small part of drug policy. All of the people who are legitimate stakeholders have a number of incommensurable concerns, and there is no reason to believe that they would weigh them similarly, even if they could individually give weight to each concern. Moreover, the consequences of different options—measured in terms of the various concerns—are almost impossible to predict with any completeness.

Brownsberger enriches and makes more difficult the problem by pushing us to take seriously the distribution of cost and benefits among different demographic groups, defined by wealth or neighborhood or ethnicity. The message that all three authors convey is that the only answer may be in decentralization to a level of decisionmaking where first-hand experience substitutes for prediction, where the differences in individual and group concerns are salient and detectable, where experiment is possible, and where change of course can more easily correct mistakes and errors of judgment. Paternalism may be essential, as the first group of authors argue. But it is conceptually and practically too difficult to be trusted to deal at a great distance with concerns as varied as those affecting drug policy.

Finally, Kleiman and Brownsberger urge us to address an issue that Jeremy Bentham addressed more than a century ago: How do we maximize the benefits of sanctions and minimize the harm that sanctions do? Caulkins and Heymann are plainly concerned about the same question as it affects almost one and a half million people arrested each year for drug offenses. Kleiman and Brownsberger are focused on heavy users, their unresponsiveness to large but uncertain and delayed sanctions, and the possibilities for tailoring sanctions much more effectively to reduce dependent use and the harms that it brings to the individual, his family, his neighborhood, and the society at large. For Caulkins and Heymann, the other side of this concern about the immorality of wasted punishment is finding a substitute for high mandatory minimum sentences.

The depth of any practical discussion of public issues depends upon the mixture of ethical concerns about "who should decide" with policy deliberation about "what is best to do." The richness of the mix depends upon whether the discussion of policy is also illuminated by clearer conceptual structures, attention to factual relationships that have not previously been adequately explored, and a depth of insight based on familiarity with what has gone before. The chapters of this book are intended to bring together these ingredients, not in the hope of solving a problem as deep and difficult as the drug problem in the United States, but in the hope of changing notions of what is most important and bringing new and useful perspectives to a problem that will be with us for the foreseeable future.

Toward a Balanced Drug-Prevention Strategy: A Conceptual Map

1

Mark H. Moore

Public discussions of drug policy have come to rely on some conventional distinctions. "Zero tolerance" policies aimed at eliminating all illicit drug use are contrasted with "harm reduction" policies designed to reduce the adverse consequences of drug use (Caulkins and Reuter 1997). Policies designed to "reduce the supply" of drugs are contrasted with those aimed at "reducing the demand" (Domestic Council Drug Abuse Task Force 1975; Rydell and Everingham 1994). Among "supply-reduction" policies, overseas efforts to eradicate crops and immobilize international trafficking networks are contrasted with efforts made at the border to interdict the flow of drugs, and with efforts to suppress street-level drug markets (Moore 1990). Among "demand-reduction" policies, distinctions are made between "prevention programs" (generally, programs designed to dissuade teenagers from using drugs; Botvin 1990) and "treatment programs" (including methadone maintenance, therapeutic communities, and 12-Step programs; Gerstein and Harwood 1990).

Such distinctions have their uses. They remind us of the varied tools available to manage the problem. They allow us to analyze the "balance" in the current portfolio of policy instruments (Office of National Drug Control Policy 1999a, 4). And, insofar as we think we know the most desirable portfolio for dealing with the drug problem, they allow us to see how close we are to that optimum (Tragler, Caulkins, and Feichtinger 1997).

Less usefully, however, these distinctions align themselves with important political ideologies. Those on the right of the political spectrum generally favor "zero tolerance" polices over "harm-reduction policies." They also favor supply reduction and drug law enforcement over prevention and treatment. Those on the political left generally favor the opposite. Often, then, the concepts are used less as analytic tools for considering the best possible combination of policies than as ideological clubs to hammer one side or the other in the apparently endless debate over drug policy.

The concept of "drug abuse prevention" is often used precisely in these ways. Fueled by the commonsense view that "an ounce of prevention is worth a pound of cure," support for drug abuse prevention is widespread. The broad enthusiasm for the general idea of prevention translates into sustained support for particular policy instruments that are conventionally described as the "prevention" component of drug abuse policy: primarily school-based programs designed to dissuade children from using drugs.[1] Those programs, in turn, build a constituency of parents, schools, and drug educators who lobby for a continued emphasis on prevention.

My purpose here is to challenge these comfortable assumptions. My aim is to clarify the concept of "drug abuse prevention" so that it can do some analytical rather than political work. More particularly, I want to distinguish an *effect* that could be called *preventive* from a *program* that is described as a *prevention program*. Using this distinction, I want to argue that supply reduction and drug law enforcement measures produce some of the most important preventive effects of current drug policy instruments. Indeed, in my view, these preventive effects provide the principal justification for relying as much as we do on these instruments (Moore 1990). In contrast, the programs that are often considered prevention programs either have little preventive effect or produce their preventive effects only in combination with other policy instruments, including drug law enforcement.

I also want to argue that drug problems often emerge as "epidemics," and that the proper balance among drug policy instruments depends on the stage of the epidemic the society confronts (Behrens 1997; Behrens and Caulkins 1997). Supply reduction and drug law enforcement instruments have a particularly important role to play at the onset of drug epidemics, while treatment programs play a more important role at later stages of the epidemic. In short, my aim is to develop and defend a different definition of drug prevention from the one that is usually relied upon, and then, using that definition, to reconsider the proper balance to maintain in our portfolio of drug policy instruments.

A Simple Analytic Model of the Drug Problem

To start, consider the simplified model of the drug "problem" presented as Figure 1.1.[2] Briefly, this model characterizes the drug problem as a commonly imagined set of *adverse consequences* of drug use. These adverse consequences affect both the drug user (damaged health, reduced economic resourcefulness, and degraded social functioning) and the wider society (crime, increased public spending).

Of course, what are commonly called the adverse consequences of drug use are, in fact, only partly caused by drug use in itself. Also implicated are the effects of individual personality, social conditions, and public policies (MacCoun and Reuter 1998). For example, the adverse health consequences of drug use on users are produced partly by the drugs themselves, but also by the fact that drugs that have been made illicit by public policy come to users in unsterile and unpredictable doses. The reduced economic resourcefulness is produced partly by the fact that drug use makes people less competent at jobs, but also by the fact our public and private policies treat drug users as unreliable employees. So, when observing the poor condition and behavior of many drug users, we must keep in mind that we are looking at the effects of personality, social structure, and public policy as well as of drug use in itself.

However important the patterns of drug use are in producing adverse consequences for users and the wider society, these patterns of use emerge from an underlying demand for drugs. Biology, individual personality, and environmental conditions shape that underlying demand. Some portion of that demand expresses itself as realized drug consumption through the operations of drug markets in which more

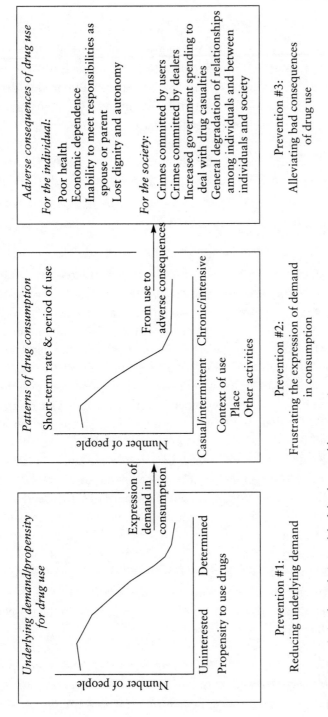

Figure 1.1. A simple analytic model of the drug problem, part 1.

or less enthusiastic demanders meet more or less cautious and greedy suppliers to sustain individual and aggregate patterns of drug use.

Note that this simple model leaves room for three different kinds of prevention policies. First, policies that reduce the underlying demand for drugs. Second, policies that make it difficult for any underlying level of demand to be expressed in sustained consumption. Third, policies that alter the relationship between any given level of drug use and the adverse individual and social consequences of that use.[3] To understand this simple model more fully, let's start with the demand for drugs.

The Underlying Demand

The underlying demand for drugs can be conceptualized as a distribution of individual propensities to use drugs.[4] In all likelihood, this distribution has the shape of a log-normal distribution as illustrated in the first panel of Figure 1.1. After all, virtually everything in life— ranging from drug use, through criminal offending and corruption in police departments, to speeding on the highway and the depth of gen- uflection in Catholic churches—seems to be distributed in this way.[5] The large number of individuals toward the left of this distribution are those who are either determined never to use drugs or disinclined to do so. The smaller (but still substantial) group in the middle would be open to drug use if the circumstances were right. The small number of people at the "right tail" would be eager to use drugs and particu- larly vulnerable to developing chronic patterns of use.

It is also plausible that individual propensities to use drugs are shaped by certain, more or less durable, individual characteristics. In- dividual propensities could start with specific biological inheritances that make each of us at least a little (and some of us highly) vulnerable to the abuse potential of drugs such as heroin and cocaine (Committee on Opportunities in Drug Abuse Research 1996). The biological en- dowments, in turn, could have been revved up or damped down by the social conditions that shaped our individual development (Com- mittee to Identify Strategies to Raise the Profile of Substance Abuse and Alcoholism Research 1997). The social conditions could have shaped our psychology (that is, our more or less unconscious drives, needs, fears, passions, moods, and so on). Or they could have shaped our knowledge of and experience with drugs (that is, our conscious, cognitive understandings of drug use and its consequences). These social conditions could act on individuals through broad factors such as the individuals' objective circumstances or the mechanisms of mass culture. Or social conditions could impress themselves on individuals through the much more intimate networks that link individuals to family, friends, or school (Jacobson and Zinberg 1975).

Presumably, changes in these social conditions could change the underlying demand for drugs among individuals and therefore the overall shape of this distribution. If an economic disaster left a large proportion of the population without hope, the individual and aggregate propensity to use drugs might increase. If family structures collapsed in ways that exposed adolescent children to even greater influence by their peers, propensities to use drugs might well increase. In effect, these social conditions could shift the whole distribution of propensities to use drugs "out" toward a wider, more intense desire to use drugs. Alternatively, these changes, operating on particular segments of the population, could affect the shape and the skew of the distribution, increasing or decreasing the difference between the median propensity to consume drugs and the propensity at the right tail of the distribution.

Obviously, if the underlying propensities to use drugs changed and everything else in this model remained constant, one would expect the patterns of drug use and the adverse consequences to change as well. Policy levers that could be used to reduce the propensities to use drugs (that is, to push the whole distribution inward, toward the origin, or to tilt the distribution so there were fewer individuals at the right tail) could be considered "primary preventive instruments." For example, if some kind of medication could be administered that would make people permanently resistant to the addictive powers of psychoactive drugs, that would constitute a primary preventive capability for drug use broadly analogous to the primary preventive impact produced by the Salk vaccine on polio. Similarly, if some kind of cognitive training could produce permanent, psychological resistance to drug use, that too could be considered a primary preventive instrument. Indeed, it is precisely the hope that relatively permanent cognitive resistance training could be provided to schoolchildren that lies at the heart of our commitment to school-based prevention programs. Because many of these programs start before students have much real experience with drugs, they must perforce be counting on being able to produce a long-lasting effect (DeJong 1987).

The Supply and Availability of Drugs

Whether the underlying demand for drugs ever gets a chance to express itself in actual drug use depends a great deal on how conveniently, reliably, and inexpensively potential users can obtain drugs. That is, the level of drug consumption depends on the supply of drugs as well as on the underlying demand. Of course, if drug users want drugs, and back up their need with money to spend, profit-motivated entrepreneurs will find a way to supply the market—at least to some degree, in some particular ways, for a particular price. But, as we will see, it is possible that all those qualifications—to some degree, in some ways, at some price—may matter. If it can be made risky for drug entrepreneurs to supply drugs, fewer entrepreneurs will enter the market. They will also behave more cautiously, and will demand more money to compensate them for the risks they are running (Moore 1977). All this will make drugs less available and more expensive than they otherwise would be. If drugs are less available and more expensive, then less of the underlying demand will be expressed in actual drug consumption. How much less depends on how risky drug dealing can be made to be (Reuter and Kleiman 1986). If the risks are low, the expressed level of drug consumption will be quite high. If, however, the risks are high, the supply of drugs may be suppressed, and with that the overall level of use—*even though the underlying demand for drugs remains constant.* To the extent, then, that burdening drug dealers discourages them from providing drugs conveniently at low prices, doing so may have an important "preventive" effect. We could call this one of the preventive *effects* of supply reduction and drug law enforcement.[6]

Later I will present the details of this argument about whether and how supply reduction and drug law enforcement might produce preventive effects. Here I simply want to indicate that the underlying *demand* for drugs differs from the observed *consumption* of drugs. Further, how much of the underlying *demand* expresses itself as *con-*

sumption depends a great deal on the available *supply* of drugs. And finally, there are many things other than the underlying *demand* to use drugs that can affect the *supply*. In short, an underlying demand for drugs can call forth a supply. But how big the supply is, and how much of the underlying demand is satisfied depends on the *supply* conditions as well as the *demand* conditions.

Patterns of Use

Given an underlying demand for drugs, and some degree of drug availability, some individuals will use drugs. But how they do so—how intensively, for how long, and in what particular contexts—will vary from one user to another. Some will never advance beyond experimentation. Others will quickly become deeply involved and stay that way for a long time. Some will be able to confine their drug use to relatively safe contexts; others will not be so disciplined and their drug use will spill over to contexts in which it is physically or socially dangerous.

Note that what I have been calling a "pattern of drug use" is a complex concept (MacCoun and Reuter 1998, 208–212). One apparently simple part of the concept focuses on drug consumption: how much is being used. The other part focuses on the context of use. But even the simple idea of drug consumption has to be divided into two distinct parts.

The first part measures the short-term rate of use: how much a user consumed in a particular episode of drug taking. This is important because it determines whether the user became intoxicated or not. In principle, one can smoke a little pot, or take a little cocaine, and suffer no more impact on judgment or physical skill than if one consumed a martini, or a cup of strong coffee. (Note: I am not saying that these drugs are equally dangerous. Indeed, one of the things that makes drugs like heroin and cocaine particularly dangerous is precisely that it seems to be hard for users to keep the use of these drugs below intoxicating levels in any given episode. Further, these drugs are particularly likely to cause people to want to reach this intoxicated state over and over again.)

The second part measures the period of time over which drug use is maintained. This is important because it tells us how addicted or dependent the user has become. Combining the two dimensions, one could describe a continuum that went from "casual, intermittent users" at one end to "intensive, chronic users" at the other. "Casual" and "intensive" refer to the *short*-term rate of consumption; "intermittent" and "chronic" refer to the period over which consumption continues.

The distinction between short-term *rate* of use and long-term *period* of use is important because some of the risks and harms of drug use are tied to the risks associated with short-term intoxication while others only emerge from long-term use. One can die of a drug overdose, or get involved in a serious crime, in a short-term burst of intensive use. One can only squander one's entire savings and destroy the trust of family and friends through sustained use.

Of course, long periods of use increase the number of reckless episodes as well. The longer one sustains use, the more chances one has to become intoxicated. But, given the nature of drug use, sustained use increases the likelihood that, in any given episode, the user will become intoxicated and use the drug in dangerous contexts. It is possible that an experienced user's growing physical tolerance and knowledge of drugs would allow him to manage his use so that there were fewer reckless episodes of intoxication than among inexperienced users. But the nature of drug use seems to be that the chronic users lose control over their drug use. Thus the long-run users may produce more reckless episodes than inexperienced users—*even when we control for the overall level of use.*

This is, in fact, what Dean Gerstein and I found when we looked closely at alcohol consumption. Intensive, long-term users not only consumed much more alcohol than others; their number of "drunk days" was also disproportional to their consumption (Moore and Gerstein 1981, 24–42). In effect, while the chronic users consumed much more alcohol over the years than intermittent users, they were also more likely than the intermittent users to drink to intoxication in any given episode. The net result is that chronic drug users get a triple whammy when compared to intermittent users: not only do they get the bad effects of reckless use, they also get the bad effects of long-term use, and they get the bad effects of large numbers of particularly reckless episodes of use! This is why many of the worst consequences of drug use are concentrated among chronic intensive users.

To be analytically helpful, a "pattern of use" should describe the social and physical context in which drugs are used as well as how intensively and how long drugs are used. The reason is that the context of drug use affects the social harms associated with drug use. With respect to medical complications, for example, a drug user experiences one set of consequences when heroin is administered through sterile needles in a hospital, and quite a different set of consequences when he administers the drug to himself on the street. With respect to family welfare, it is one thing for an unmarried Wall Street yuppie with significant personal and family resources to become involved with cocaine; it is quite another for a pregnant young woman with no resources to do so. The consequences to the first user will be handled largely within private institutions relying on private resources. The consequences to the second user will, in all likelihood, spread from the mother to the child, and from the family to the broader society (Besharov 1994). The point is that the activities that are paired with drug use, and the social position of the drug user, affect the magnitude and character of the individual and social harms associated with drug use.

Insofar as the different patterns of drug use produce different social consequences, policymakers have an opportunity to prevent some bad consequences of drug use by discouraging dangerous patterns of use. For example, if we provided oral doses of methadone as a substitute for intravenous use of heroin, we could reduce the number of crimes committed by drug users and increase their level of employment. Or, if we distributed clean needles to drug users, we might be able to reduce the users' rate of septicemia or AIDS. Or, if we provided drug counseling in employment contexts, we might be able to change the relationship between drug use and unemployment. Such interventions are not designed to eliminate drug consumption; they are designed to change some part of the pattern of drug use that is causing the adverse social consequences.

The difficulty with such approaches is that we are not sure what the relationship is between relatively benign patterns of use and malignant patterns of use. If the relatively benign patterns develop into the relatively malignant patterns at a certain, unchangeable rate, then we cannot reduce the relatively malignant patterns without reducing the relatively benign patterns. This concern is part of what justifies commitments to "zero tolerance" policies: we can't afford to have any drug use, because the minor drug use will beget the serious drug use.

It is not hard to imagine mechanisms that might link relatively benign patterns of drug use to malignant patterns. If, for example, a relatively constant proportion of casual, intermittent users got swept up in the addictive and dependence-producing power of heroin and cocaine, then the amount of chronic, intensive use might be a direct function of the amount of casual, intermittent use. Or, if the relative success of drug users in benign patterns advertised the apparent safety of drug use, unsuspecting individuals with high degrees of vulnerability might be drawn into drug use and find themselves trapped. Or it may be that the high levels of use sustained by chronic, intensive users supply the core financing that supports drug markets, which then become relatively accessible to all.

The point is simply this: to the extent that benign patterns of use tend to increase the risk of advancing to malignant patterns of use, society might decide to treat the benign patterns not as tolerable behavior but instead as a "risk factor" for malignant patterns. As such, the benign patterns might become important targets of prevention efforts along with the malignant patterns. Or, if society's principal concern was with the malignant patterns, we might concentrate on finding prevention instruments that were specific to reducing the malignant patterns, leaving the benign patterns untouched.

Harms and Adverse Consequences

The patterns of use are linked to a set of *adverse consequences* of drug use that constitute the core of the drug problem. These consequences can accrue to, and be evaluated by, individual drug users. For example, users may experience more or less disabling health consequences, and may feel more or less satisfaction with their current drug-using patterns. Alternatively, the adverse consequences may accrue to, and be evaluated by, society at large. For example, drug users may commit crimes, and those crimes may affect both the individual victims and the wider society. Analytically, one could think of the harms and adverse consequences (as well as some benefits) as emerging probabilistically from any given aggregate level of drug use, distributed across a particular set of patterns. Thus an underlying propensity to use drugs, expressed through an existing market for drugs, emerges as an aggregate distribution of use patterns. The use patterns, in turn, result in an observed set of harms and adverse consequences.

As noted above, however, some particular features of patterns of use may be particularly important in linking any given level of consumption to any particular adverse consequence. For example, some of the most important adverse health consequences of drug use (such as septicemia or the spread of AIDS) may be linked to the use of borrowed, dirty needles to administer the drug—a risk common among street-level heroin addicts, less common among those who smoke crack. Or crime and child abuse may be linked more to poor drug users than to rich ones simply because the wealth of the rich insulates them from the conditions that necessitate these crimes among the poor. The rich can loot their own bank accounts rather than their neighbors' wallets, and can purchase child care for those days when they feel they can't cope.

Insofar as there are some separate causal mechanisms that link patterns of use to adverse consequences, these, too, can become the focus of prevention instruments. We can make the world more or less safe—both physically and socially—for those who use drugs in particular use patterns. We can choose to provide clean needles to drug users in the hope of changing the relationship between drug use and health consequences. We can provide cocaine-addicted mothers with combinations of support and discipline, and through such interventions alter the relationship between cocaine use and child neglect and abuse. Policies that change the relationship between patterns of drug use on the one hand and adverse consequences on the other can be called "tertiary" prevention policies.

The Environment

So far I have emphasized the way desires or propensities to use drugs "go through" to adverse consequences of drug use via drug consumption organized in various patterns of use. An obvious objection to this view is that it places far too much emphasis on the underlying demand. It ignores the impact of the environment or social conditions on the demand for drugs. And it misses the way social conditions transform relatively benign patterns of drug use into events that produce serious adverse consequences. At the extreme, some would argue that there wouldn't be much consumption of drugs if social conditions were more prosperous or more just, or if there were no financial profit in the illicit trade. Others would argue that what appear to be adverse consequences of drug use are really expressions of broader individual pathologies created by an unfair society.

These criticisms are apt. Figure 1.2 attempts to accommodate them by showing an important role for the social environment as well as for underlying demand and its expression through patterns of use to adverse consequences. The figure suggests that the broader social environment influences the size and shape of the drug problem in three important ways.

First, as noted above, the environment and social conditions are important in what might be called the *background* of both the individual propensities to use drugs and the aggregate distribution of these propensities. If society has a significant amount of poverty, racial discrimination, and family deterioration as environmental conditions, those conditions might well affect the location and shape of the underlying propensities to use drugs. In fact, one could easily imagine that these effects could be explosive in their impact: that a society with a certain level of these structural conditions might be particularly vulnerable to an epidemic of drug use in the same way that a population weakened by malnutrition might be vulnerable to a flu epidemic.

Second, environmental and social conditions may also be very much in the *foreground* of the drug problem. The social conditions in which individuals find themselves—how many of their close friends and relatives use drugs, how conveniently available drugs are, what the meaning of drug use is in their local milieu—can all affect the likelihood that an underlying individual propensity to use drugs will be expressed in a particular pattern of use.

Note that the distinction between *background* and *foreground* conditions is based on two key characteristics. One is time: a factor is in the background when it happened in the past and has accumulated

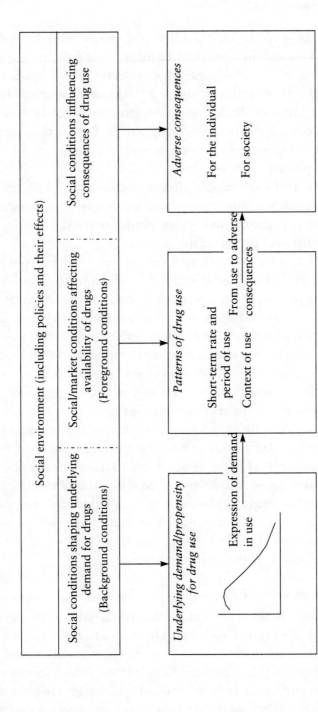

Figure 1.2. A simple analytic model of the drug problem, part 2.

within the experience of individuals or the shared experience of a community or society. In contrast, a factor is in the foreground when it is a condition an individual currently confronts. The second distinction is linked to the way background and foreground conditions operate on human behavior. Background conditions influence one's motivations and knowledge—the capital one carries around within oneself. Foreground conditions present themselves to individuals as opportunities to be exploited or neglected.

In the context of our simple model, background social conditions affect the propensity to use. Foreground social conditions affect the likelihood that a particular underlying propensity to use will be expressed in a particular pattern of use.

Third, the social environment operates not only on levels and patterns of drug use but also on the causal mechanisms that transform any given pattern of drug use into adverse social consequences. If I'm a drug user and can't find a legitimate job that fits well with my drug use, I'll end up as a criminal offender. If the crowd with whom I smoke crack likes to pair that activity with unprotected sex, I face a greater risk of contracting AIDS than if my drug-using crowd uses LSD for lonely introspection. In this sense, my environment exacerbates the adverse consequences of using drugs.

In this model, then, the broader social environment is an important factor shaping the size and character of the drug problem via three different mechanisms: (1) by producing important environmental influences on the location and shape of the underlying distribution of propensities to use drugs; (2) by influencing whether and how those propensities are translated into particular individual and aggregate patterns of use; and (3) by influencing how those patterns of use are translated into levels of adverse consequences.

Policies as Environmental Factors

The simple model is also vulnerable to the criticism that it ignores the fact that many of the most important observed adverse consequences of drug use emerge not from drug use in itself but as unintended effects of drug policies (MacCoun and Reuter 1998). Thus the only reason drug users end up committing property and violent crimes is that laws prohibiting the sale of drugs make the drugs expensive and not conveniently available. Since not all drug users can become highly paid consultants working flexible hours, some must turn to crime to maintain their habits. Or the only reason drug users become so unhealthy is that drugs sold in illicit markets cannot be quality controlled and are apt to be unpredictable as to dose and loaded up with dangerous contaminants.

This criticism, too, is apt. One way to deal with it is to treat the broad social conditions that affect the drug problem as inclusive of the conditions created by drug and other social policies. Thus the current level of poverty and racial discrimination in labor markets could be seen as at least partly a consequence of failed policies in these areas. Economic and social conditions within neighborhoods could be seen as consequences of economic development policies.

Of more immediate concern, perhaps, is that the character of local drug distribution systems and the markets they help to sustain—how big, how visible, how easily accessed, how expensive, how risky, and so on—can and should be seen as the result of policies toward drug trafficking. The foreground factors described above may be strongly influenced by drug enforcement activities of one kind or another (Moore 1990; Chaiken 1988).

Equally important is the idea that drug policies can affect the attitudes of both the wider public and the immediate neighbors of drug users. Those attitudes, in turn, become part of the foreground social conditions that drug users confront. A society largely committed to "zero tolerance" may succeed in discouraging drug use among many; but for those who use drugs despite the intolerance, the consequences will be much worse. Their drug use will result in social disapprobation, loss of employment, and so on. Such sanctions may, in the long run, help the committed users abandon their drug use through the mechanism of specific deterrence. Or they may simply inflict a loss on the drug users and the rest of us without producing any real deterrent effects.

Prevention Policies

With this simple model of the drug abuse problem, it is possible to be more precise about what we might mean by drug prevention policies.

Prevention as an Effect or as a Kind of Policy?

The first question to be answered is whether we want to define prevention policies in terms of their *effects* or in terms of a particular *target* or *mode of operation*. Arguably, a prevention policy could be any policy designed to produce, or actually producing, an effect on either overall levels of drug use or adverse consequences. This broad definition would certainly embrace treatment policies. It might also include supply reduction and drug law enforcement options. In fact, this definition of drug prevention is so broad that it excludes no important drug policy instruments.

A more restrictive definition would limit prevention programs to those which operate on specific parts of the drug abuse problem in particular ways (Polich et al. 1984). For example, we could limit drug prevention policies to those designed to prevent persons who have never used drugs from initiating use. This definition would exclude treatment programs that seek to prevent future use by persuading current users to give up their drug use. And it would exclude early intervention programs that seek to discourage experimental users from advancing to more chronic, intensive drug use.

Or we could narrow the definition still further and limit drug prevention policies to those which aim to prevent the initiation of drug use by developing decisionmaking and peer-resistance skills among teenagers. Indeed, this last definition is what "prevention programs" ordinarily mean in drug policy debates. Such prevention programs can be based on mass media or on more intimate and intensive forms of communication. And they can be paired with various kinds of additional activities such as health education or after-school recreation programs. But the core idea is that prevention programs are information programs designed to dissuade those not now using drugs from beginning to do so (Polich et al. 1984).

Obviously, there are enormous differences among these definitions of drug prevention policies. In principle there is nothing wrong in having several different definitions of drug prevention policies. The only practical difficulty comes if we assume, on a commonsense basis, that any effective drug policy should have a preventive component, and then assume that that commonsense intuition justifies expenditures on the particular kinds of prevention programs included in the second definition without testing them against the power of other instruments to produce the same preventive results (Caulkins et al. 1998).

Note that there are two analytic failures here. One is to assume that "prevention" (however defined) is self-evidently a valuable component of drug policy—"an ounce of prevention is worth a pound of cure"—when it is by no means clear that this is true. The second is to assume that whatever value prevention policies may have is realized through the use of a particular kind of policy instrument: namely programs directed at people who are not yet users, operating through the mechanisms of persuasion to reduce the likelihood of future use. Both assumptions *may* be true, but their truth cannot and should not be taken as given. If we are interested in drug abuse prevention on *prima facie* grounds, we should at least explore the relative effectiveness of different instruments in achieving the desired effect.

Prevention of What?

The second question to be answered is about the goal of drug prevention policies. Is the goal (1) to reduce drug use of any kind, (2) to reduce the patterns of drug use that are particularly likely to produce adverse consequences, or (3) to reduce the adverse consequences of drug use without worrying too much about the underlying levels or patterns of use (Caulkins and Reuter 1997)? This is a very important question. The reason is that programs designed to prevent all drug use may have a negative impact on the goal of reducing adverse consequences, while those designed to reduce adverse consequences may have a negative impact on the goal of reducing all drug use.

For example, if society wanted to discourage drug use in general or particular patterns of drug use, it could decide to achieve this goal by stigmatizing particular patterns of drug use. It could pass laws prohibiting certain patterns of use. Or it could mobilize cultural antipathies to using certain kinds of drugs in particular ways. If society succeeded in these efforts, it would create a social environment hostile to those who used drugs despite the prohibition or stigma. That hostility, in turn, would produce consequences that were adverse not only to the drug users themselves but possibly also to the society at large. If employers react to drug use by firing drug users, the fired employees are adversely affected. But society is adversely affected as well if it has to pay the unemployment compensation, or endure the reduced productivity, or suffer through the crimes that the unemployed users will commit. If wives react to drug use by throwing their husbands out, or parents react the same way to drug-using teenagers, that, too, can be bad not only for the drug-using husbands and teenagers but also for the wider society.

Conversely, if society wanted to focus on reducing the harms of drug use, without worrying so much about underlying levels of consumption, it might adopt policies designed to make the world a safer place in which to be intoxicated or drug dependent. Thus it might want to increase tolerance of drug use—particularly of forms of use that did not seem to create bad consequences for the user or the wider society. We might even want to change the environment in ways that would make it safer to be intoxicated: by, for example, reducing the availability of weapons or making mattresses that were less likely to catch fire when burning cigarettes fell from sleeping hands. This might protect drug users from some of the bad consequences of their use. But for precisely these reasons, it might very well increase overall levels of use. Since the penalties for use had been reduced, reasons for resisting use would have been attenuated.

The tension between reducing drug use in itself and reducing the bad consequences of drug use seems intrinsic (Kleiman 1992). The reason is that if society's goal is to reduce drug use, it wants to use the bad consequences of drug use to help discourage the practice. In fact, it doesn't want to wait for the naturally occurring bad consequences of drug use to show up sometime in the future for drug users; it wants to construct quicker and more certain bad consequences of drug use to warn users of the real harms of drug use (Musto 1973). In doing so, it may reduce overall drug use, but only at the cost of increasing the adverse consequences to those who continue to use. When society comes to review its drug policies, then, what will be apparent is the impact of the policies on those who were not dissuaded from use. What will be less apparent is the impact of the policies on dissuading others from using.

On the other hand, if society's goal is to reduce the adverse consequences of drug use and not consumption (let alone the underlying propensity to use drugs), then it may deliberately decide to insulate drug users from many of the consequences of drug use. Doing so may reduce the harms experienced by drug users. But precisely for that reason, the same policies may increase the total number of users in any given use pattern.

Whether it makes sense to focus preventive efforts on drug use in itself or on its adverse consequences depends on different factors, about which people make quite different assumptions. Three key assumptions are: (1) how responsive drug use is to difficulty in obtaining drugs or adverse consequences of drug use; (2) how bad drug use in itself would be once shorn of the iatrogenic effects of policies designed to discourage drug use; and (3) how likely it is that drug users, given some starting level of use, will advance to dangerous patterns of use.

If one assumes that individuals are naturally destined to use drugs or not, and that little in their actual experience with drugs will affect their fate, then one naturally favors "harm reduction" policies over "use reduction" policies. The reason is that, under these assumptions, there is little that society can do to reduce consumption, therefore little price to be paid for making the world a safe place in which to be intoxicated or drug dependent. (This assumption may make sense, but to be consistent, one must recognize that this claim renders treatment and the more limited forms of prevention doubtful, since they depend on being able to dissuade users from using drugs.)

Similarly, if one assumes that most of the observed bad consequences of drug use—poor health, unemployment, crime, and so on—result from efforts to make drugs unavailable and unattractive to users rather than from drug use in itself, then one will favor harm-reduction policies over those designed to reduce consumption. The reason is that since all the burden of drug use comes from the adverse consequences produced by policies designed to reduce use, we can relax those policies and get the benefits of reducing adverse consequences while not increasing the total number of users.

And, if one assumes that very few users who are now using drugs in relatively harmless patterns will advance to dangerous patterns of use, then one will, once again, favor harm-reduction policies over use-reduction policies. The reason, again, is that there is little to be gained (and some important losses to be incurred) by trying to prevent people from advancing to dangerous use patterns.

Alternatively, if one makes the opposite assumptions—that consumption of drugs is responsive to social stigma, to difficulty in purchasing drugs, to real adverse consequences of using drugs; that many of the bad consequences of drug use result from using drugs, not just from the artificially constructed hazards; and that seemingly harmless patterns of drug use elevate the risk that users will advance to more dangerous patterns of use—then one tends to take a more benign view of policies designed to prevent drug use, even if these increase the adverse consequences of drug use for those who are not dissuaded. It is here that the sharpest debates about drug policy occur.

Points of Intervention

It is useful, in talking about drug prevention policies, to get past these fundamental issues and to look more closely at an array of drug prevention policy instruments that are targeted at different points of intervention. Five useful distinctions can be made.

As noted above, the first kind of prevention policy could be characterized as "primary prevention." I will define these as policies that focus on the environmental conditions that affect the underlying propensities to use drugs. This could include social policies aimed at reducing poverty and racial discrimination, increasing employment opportunities, or strengthening the capacities of families to care for their children. For the most part, these efforts are not thought of as drug policy but as more fundamental social policy. Their effect on preventing drug use is secondary to their most important justification, which is to alter damaging social conditions.

The second kind of prevention policies might be called "secondary prevention." These are designed to affect the milieu within which potential and current experimental users interact with one another. This includes the array of after-school activities available to teenagers, the prevailing views about drug use held within different teen subcultures, and so on. The aim of these policies is to reduce the social supports to and the enabling conditions of drug use among particularly vulnerable populations. These are what are most commonly viewed as drug prevention policies.

The third kind of prevention policies might also be considered "secondary prevention" programs, but instead of working on the demand side of the market, they work on the supply side. It is here that many supply-reduction efforts—ranging from eradication programs in source countries, through interdiction, to street-level drug enforcement—can have their preventive effects. Insofar as these programs succeed in making it harder, more expensive, and more dangerous for users to gain access to drugs, they may help to discourage new users from beginning to use and casual users from advancing to more serious use patterns. They may also help create conditions under which those in serious use patterns seek treatment on their own or are exposed to criminal justice interventions that require them to seek treatment.

A fourth kind of prevention policy could be considered "tertiary prevention." Those policies are designed to break the connection between any given pattern of use and the adverse consequence—to reduce the adverse consequences associated with any given level of use.

It is worth noting that what are commonly called drug abuse prevention programs are really exploiting only one of these possible points of intervention: the milieu of social supports and enabling conditions surrounding those not-yet-users judged to be particularly vulnerable to drug use. Within this family of policies we can distinguish between policies that operate through mass instruments such as advertising and those which operate through more tailored, intimate instruments such as drug resistance education or individualized drug counseling. These programs can focus on drug use specifically or on health and responsibility more generally. They can be designed to influence individual knowledge and cognition or to develop individuals' resistance to peer influences. While there are many variants of this kind of drug prevention program, they all can usefully be seen as one broad family of preventive interventions. Thus they must compete with other forms of prevention efforts—notably with primary prevention, with secondary prevention focused on drug markets, and with tertiary prevention designed to break the link between drug use and adverse consequences (such as needle exchange programs). In the remainder of this chapter, I would like to develop the idea of supply-reduction and drug law enforcement policies as important drug prevention policies—not simply as expressive instruments of a zero tolerance policy.

Supply Reduction and Drug Law Enforcement

Many people have come to believe that supply-reduction and drug law enforcement efforts have little impact on the supply of drugs, and therefore little impact on the overall level of drug use. This is possible. And given the enormous direct and indirect costs of such efforts, this possibility should loom large in discussions of drug policies. But arguing the theoretical possibility is very different from imagining that one has a lever that could end legal restrictions against the production and distribution of drugs such as cocaine and heroin, and deciding to go ahead and push the lever. Before pushing the lever, one might want to consider the following observations and facts.

First, it is worth remembering that prohibiting the production and distribution of drugs such as heroin and cocaine does significantly burden drug entrepreneurs. It exposes them to the threat of arrest and long prison terms. And, despite the claim that imprisonment matters little or is even viewed positively by young drug dealers, it seems unlikely that drug dealers would prefer to be in prison rather than on the street (Reuter, MacCoun, and Murphy 1990). Perhaps more important, making drug trafficking illegal denies drug dealers the protection of the law, and thereby exposes them to rip-offs and violence at the hands of other dealers and criminals (Moore 1990). There may well be many young men who are willing to face these risks. This means that drug law enforcement policies cannot totally eliminate drug dealing. But it is unlikely that the number of those willing to be drug dealers facing these risks is greater than the number of those who would be willing to deal drugs if doing so were legal. If there are fewer dealers, the supply will be less, and the amount of consumption will be less than it otherwise would be. This is fundamental economic theory.

Second, if dealers are exposed to threats from law enforcement agents and other criminals but nonetheless decide to continue dealing drugs, they will operate in ways that are designed to (1) reduce the risks they face and (2) compensate them for the risks they cannot reduce (Moore 1977). One way they will reduce their risks is to limit their dealing to people they trust. This means that they will prefer to deal with those who are already using drugs rather than run the risk of recruiting new users. The way they will compensate themselves for the risk of dealing drugs is to raise prices. The net effect of both these responses will be to increase the "effective price" of drugs to users, and perhaps particularly to new users. By the effective price I mean the total amount of time, effort, money, risk, and other kinds of inconvenience customers must endure to purchase drugs.

The effective price may differ from user to user. Experienced drug users may well face lower effective prices than less experienced users. Inexperienced users in neighborhoods where drugs are commonly used will face lower effective prices than those in neighborhoods where drugs are less commonly available. Moreover, the effective price will never be entirely prohibitive. Given enough money and effort, one can probably find drugs to buy even if one looks like an undercover narcotics agent, let alone a drug addict.

But all these points mean is that some drugs will continue to be sold—an unsurprising conclusion. Those at the right tail of the distribution of propensities to use drugs will find some way to score. This does not mean that the aggregate amount of drugs sold will be the same as if the effective price were uniform and low. At some (plausibly achievable) high level of effective prices, some in the middle of the distribution of the propensity to consume will be discouraged from doing so. And that is an effect that might be worth counting as prevention—particularly if some of those who are discouraged from using are young people who have limited experience with drugs. High effective prices to them should create a large negative response (because their elasticity of demand with respect to changes in the effective price of drugs is very high).

So far I have been making primarily theoretical arguments for considering supply-reduction and drug law enforcement policies as potentially important in preventing drug use. I have not presented any empirical evidence to show that the effects I am claiming actually exist or are large enough to matter. The only empirical evidence I can present is the following.

First, on the question of whether supply-reduction efforts can succeed in raising the effective price of drugs, it is worth comparing the prices of illegal drugs to close substitutes that are legal. Table 1.1 compares the price of heroin in illicit markets with that of methadone in licit markets, and the price of cocaine in illicit markets with that of

Table 1.1 Illegal versus legal drug prices

Drug	Current retail price	Estimated legal price	Ratio
Heroin (pure gram)	$2,280	$30–35	70:1
Cocaine (pure gram)	$143	$15–20	8:1
Marijuana (cigarette)	95¢	6–7¢	15:1

Source: Moore 1990, 124. Legal heroin price estimated from prevailing legal prices for morphine and methadone. Legal cocaine price estimated from prevailing prices for cocaine. Legal marijuana price estimated from prevailing prices of tobacco cigarettes.

cocaine in licit markets.[7] It is clear from this table that there is something about making drugs illegal that makes them expensive and probably less conveniently available as well. Illicit heroin is 70 times more expensive than methadone; and illicit cocaine is 8 times more expensive than legal cocaine (even though legal cocaine has a small and specialized demand, and therefore may be much more expensive in legal markets now than it would be under more liberal regimes).

Second, one might imagine that these changes in price would have little impact on committed drug users. That might well be true. But one has to keep in mind that the goal is to prevent and reduce drug use among less committed users as well as committed ones. Further, price increases significantly less than these have been shown to reduce consumption of alcohol and cigarettes among alcoholics and two-pack-a-day smokers as well as among less committed users. Part of the reason is that those at the right tail of the distribution consume drugs so intensively that small changes in price translate into large new expenditure requirements that are not easy to meet. That seems to make a difference even to highly committed users.

Considering the issue more empirically, a National Academy of Sciences panel recently established a range of estimates for the price elasticity of the demand for cocaine ranging from -0.38 to -1.00 or even more (Manski, Pepper, and Thomas 1999, 26). These numbers suggest that if we let the price of cocaine fall by a factor of 10 (which would be roughly the effect of allowing the drugs to fall to their current legal price), we could expect cocaine consumption to increase between 380 and 1,000 percent—a nontrivial result! Such numbers should not be taken too seriously, but they do remind us that drug consumption could be relatively inelastic and quite unresponsive to price and still be strongly influenced if the change in price is large enough. It may be important, then, that the combination of making drugs illegal and enforcing the laws against them seems to be able to drive up the price by 1,000 percent.

Third, while it is hard to determine whether increases or decreases in drug consumption are produced by changes in demand, or changes in supply, or some combination of the two, there are some conditions involving changes in price and consumption that produce unequivocal evidence of the impact of reductions in supply (Moore 1990). If, for example, prices are rising as consumption is falling, it is unambiguous that the supply of drugs has diminished. On the other hand, if prices are falling while consumption is increasing, it is unambiguous that supply has increased. Applying this simple diagnostic test to the past few decades of experience with American drug markets, one can conclude that there have been three supply-reduction successes and one remarkable supply-reduction failure. The three successes involved heroin in the late sixties and early seventies, heroin again in the late seventies, and marijuana in the eighties. The remarkable failure was the worst drug epidemic the country has faced: cocaine that surged in the late eighties. This failure was to some degree inexplicable. It is as if the supply system kept growing beyond the capacity of supply-reduction efforts to inhibit it. Viewed from this perspective, the supply-reduction efforts may have produced some beneficial results even as the cocaine epidemic was spreading. But they were simply not enough to stem the tide.

Drug Epidemics, Supply Reduction, and Drug Law Enforcement

As noted above, whether one considers policies focused on supply reduction and drug law enforcement effective preventive instruments depends a great deal on one's assumptions about whether they can be effective in standing in the way of underlying propensities to use drugs expressing themselves in actual drug use. This is a key issue. The use of the imagery of "drug epidemics" is related to this question, and is therefore worth some independent consideration.

The public health community makes an important distinction between conditions considered "endemic" and those considered "epidemic." The distinction is based on the relationship between current conditions and what is expected. If a disease is occurring at levels within a normal, expected range, the problem is said to be "endemic." If, on the other hand, a problem is occurring at an unexpected, elevated rate, it is considered "epidemic."

The idea of an epidemic is often confused with the idea that there are some important causal mechanisms at work that are producing nonlinear increases in the problem. There are many contagious or other nonlinear processes that could lie behind epidemics of drug use (Hunt and Chambers 1976).

Many analysts consider drug use in the United States an endemic rather than an epidemic problem (National Commission on Marihuana and Drug Abuse 1973). These analysts tend to look at the use of many different intoxicants, including alcohol, tobacco, and marijuana, and conclude that the overall level of drug use has not changed much over time. In this sense, the drug problem seems endemic. There may be some local epidemics of drug use associated with particular fads or the emergence of some kind of specialized local supply. But usually these are just blips in a relatively constant overall pattern of drug use.

Other analysts, however, would say that while America may have endemic drug problems associated with alcohol, tobacco, and marijuana, America has also experienced several important epidemics of drug use over the last few decades. In this view, America faced a serious epidemic of heroin use in the late sixties and early seventies, which abated in the mid-seventies and then reappeared in the late seventies. And it faced an even more serious epidemic of cocaine use that appeared in the early eighties and worsened throughout that decade, becoming an epidemic of use of crack as well as powder cocaine. Arguably, the cocaine epidemic was by far the worst of these epidemics. It affected many more people than the heroin epidemic. It crossed class boundaries in ways that the heroin epidemic did not. And perhaps most important, it involved women in large numbers as well as men. The social consequences of this epidemic showed up in all parts of the society—in labor markets, in welfare and child-protection systems, in criminal justice agencies, and in medical institutions.

There are several important implications of thinking of drug abuse as an epidemic rather than an endemic problem. First, it makes it seem as though the problem may be solvable. If one can find the proximate cause of the epidemic, one may be able to intervene to stop it.

Second, it stimulates a search for the immediate cause, and for ways to bring that cause under control. Here there are many candidates. One idea is that drug use is spread by cultural trends aided and abetted by the mass media. Another is that drug use is spread through interconnected networks of peers vouching for the pleasure and safety of the experience (Hunt and Chambers 1976). In these accounts, one characteristic that allows the epidemic to spread is the fact that the long-term adverse consequences of drug use have not yet appeared. Drug use looks safe. Once the epidemic has gone on long enough to produce chronic intensive users, with all their adverse consequences, the epidemic will have run its course. The society will learn for itself that drug use is bad (Musto 1973).

Note that these familiar accounts focus on demand-side explanations. But one could also explain the emergence and abatement of drug epidemics in supply-side terms. This explanation would put a lot of the explanatory weight on the development of illicit distribution channels. Indeed, one extreme version of this theory sees the entire explanation for drug epidemics in changes in supply. This view holds that the underlying demand for drugs in a society doesn't change very much or very fast. It is fixed at a relatively high level. It is fixed there partly as a consequence of inherited biological vulnerabilities to drugs such as heroin and cocaine, and partly as a consequence of social conditions such as poverty and discrimination that make us vulnerable to drug epidemics. In this conception, all societies are vulnerable to drug epidemics all the time on the demand side.

What ignites an epidemic at a particular place and time—what transforms that vulnerability into a painful reality—is not, then, changes on the demand side. It is, instead, changes on the supply side. Once the epidemic occurs, one can say that it was caused by an underlying high level of demand and the emergence of a supply system. But what made the epidemic happen at a particular place and time was the change in the supply conditions, not a change in the underlying demand.

This view is given some credence by the fact that the earliest signs of a coming epidemic appear on the supply side. It is not usually that poverty suddenly deepens or discrimination becomes more virulent. It is that some bad guys start showing up with suitcases full of illicit drugs. If this analysis is correct, then one can treat the changes in supply conditions as an important proximate cause of drug epidemics.

The third important implication of thinking of the drug problem as an epidemic is that what is considered an appropriate balance among drug policy instruments may differ depending upon the stage of the epidemic (Behrens 1997). At the early stages of an epidemic it will make sense to emphasize supply reduction and drug law enforcement to minimize the spread of the epidemic. At this stage it may also make sense to invest heavily in secondary prevention policies focused on those at risk of drug use to reduce the number of susceptibles, and to deny the developing drug markets consumers who can fuel their continued growth. The point is that an all-out effort should be made to halt the spread of the epidemic in its early days. Later in the epidemic, when the real consequences of drug use have become more apparent to all, and when the society has accumulated a large number of casualties who need sustained attention, the balance of drug policy should shift toward treatment rather than supply reduction or secondary prevention. It is then that society must work on trying to reduce the adverse consequences of drug use for those who became involved while the epidemic was spreading.

Conclusion

No doubt prevention must be an important part of drug policy. But in deciding what role prevention must play, it is important to be clearer than we have been in defining what we mean by prevention, and more accurate in our attribution of preventive effects to particular policy instruments. We might all think that the best way to solve the drug problem is through primary preventive efforts designed to eliminate social conditions—such as poverty and racial discrimination—that influence the underlying propensities for using drugs. But it is worth keeping in mind that these important efforts to prevent drug use cannot be easily distinguished from more general social policies that are justified in their own right—not primarily as means to prevent drug use.

We might also find some important uses for secondary prevention policies focused more narrowly on the attitudes, social supports, and conditions surrounding potential drug users. But it is possible that the most important drug prevention effects are achieved through supply reduction and drug law enforcement efforts. Indeed, these instruments may be particularly valuable in preventing the spread of drug-abuse epidemics when they break out. These policies always have the undesirable consequences of worsening the condition of those who continue to use drugs despite the stigma and the practical difficulties, to the misfortune not only of the users themselves but also of the rest of society. Consequently, these policies may be usefully combined with "tertiary prevention policies" such as treatment programs that are designed not only to reduce consumption among committed users but also to break the link between their continued use and their adverse individual and social consequences.

From this perspective, what has often been viewed as an overreliance on drug law enforcement and an underinvestment in preventive measures is turned on its head: it is precisely our interest in preventing drug use that counsels the continued use of drug law enforcement as a preventive instrument.

Notes

1. The federal government spends $2.08 billion, or about 12 percent of its overall drug budget, on these programs (Office of National Drug Control Policy 1999b). On these programs see Jacobson and Zinberg 1975; Polich et al. 1984; Botvin 1990.
2. For a similar model and conceptual framework used in the analysis of alcohol prevention policies, see Moore and Gerstein 1981.
3. These kinds of policies correspond roughly to the conventional public health distinctions among "primary," "secondary," and "tertiary" preventive efforts. Primary prevention seeks to alter the general conditions that

cause a public health problem to emerge. Secondary prevention seeks to reduce risks to high-risk populations by creating obstacles to the development or spread of a health problem. Tertiary prevention seeks to reduce the seriousness of the consequences of the health problem. See also Polich et al. 1984, 117–120.

4. A similar idea—that there are relatively stable, underlying propensities to engage in disapproved behavior distributed across a broad range—has gained some currency in the exploration of criminal offending (see Blumstein et al. 1986) and the use of alcohol (see Moore and Gerstein 1981).

5. This hypothesis was first advanced in 1934; see Allport 1934.

6. On elasticity of demand and the elastic demand of new users see Moore 1973.

7. Because cocaine, unlike heroin, has legitimate medical uses, it is classified in Schedule II of the Controlled Substances Act and may be sold for limited medical purposes. It is used as a topical anesthetic in dentistry.

References

Allport, Floyd H. 1934. "The J-Curve Hypothesis of Conforming Behavior." *Journal of Social Psychology* 5: 141–183.

Behrens, Doris. 1997. "Optimal Control of Drug Epidemics: Prevent and Treat—But Not at the Same Time." Vienna University of Technology.

Behrens, Doris, and Jonathan P. Caulkins. 1997. "A Dynamic Model of Drug Initiation: Implications for Treatment and Drug Control." Vienna University of Technology.

Besharov, Douglas J., ed. 1994. *When Drug Addicts Have Children: Re-Orienting Child Welfare's Response.* Washington: American Enterprise Institute.

Blumstein, Alfred, et al., eds. 1986. *Criminal Careers and Career Criminals,* vol. 1. Washington: National Academy of Sciences Press.

Botvin, G. J. 1990. "Substance Abuse Prevention: Theory, Practice and Evidence." In Michael Tonry and James Q. Wilson, eds., *Drugs and Crime: Crime and Justice,* vol. 13. Chicago: University of Chicago Press.

Caulkins, Jonathan P., and Peter Reuter. 1997. "Setting Goals for Drug Policy: Harm Reduction or Use Reduction." 92: 1143–50.

Caulkins, J. P., et al. 1998. "The Cost-Effectiveness of School-Based Drug Prevention Programs: An Ounce of Prevention, a Pound of Uncertainty." Santa Monica: Rand.

Chaiken, Marcia R., ed. 1988. *Street Level Drug Enforcement: Examining the Issues.* Washington: Department of Justice, National Institute of Justice.

Committee to Identify Strategies to Raise the Profile of Substance Abuse and Alcoholism Research. 1997. "Dispelling Myths about Addiction: Strategies to Increase Understanding and Strengthen Research." Washington: National Academy of Sciences.

Committee on Opportunities in Drug Abuse Research. 1996. "Pathways of Addiction: Opportunities in Drug Abuse Research." Washington: National Academy of Sciences.

DeJong, William. 1987. "Arresting the Demand for Drugs: Police and School Partnerships to Prevent Drug Abuse." Washington: Department of Justice, National Institute of Justice.

Domestic Council Drug Abuse Task Force. 1975. "White Paper on Drug Abuse." Washington: Executive Office of the President.

Ellickson, Phyllis, and Robert M. Bell. 1990. "Prospects for Preventing Drug Use among Young Adolescents." Santa Monica: Rand.

Ellickson, Phyllis, et al. 1988. "Designing and Implementing Project ALERT: A Smoking and Drug Prevention Experiment." Santa Monica: Rand.

Gerstein, Dean R., and Henrick Harwood, eds. 1990. *Treating Drug Problems,* vol. 1: *A Study of the Effectiveness and Financing of Public and Private Drug Treatment Systems.* Washington: National Academy of Sciences Press.

Hunt, Leon Gibson, and Carl D. Chambers. 1976. *The Heroin Epidemics.* Sociomedical Science Series. New York: Spectrum Publications.

Jacobson, Richard, and Norman E. Zinberg. 1975. "The Social Basis of Drug Abuse Prevention." Drug Abuse Council, 1975.

Kleiman, Mark A. R. 1992. *Against Excess: Drug Policy for Results.* New York: Basic Books.

MacCoun, Robert, and Peter Reuter. 1998. "Drug Control." In Michael Tonry, ed., *The Handbook of Crime and Punishment.* New York: Oxford University Press.

Manski, Charles F., John V. Pepper, and Yonette Thomas. 1999. "Assessment of Two Cost-Effectiveness Studies on Cocaine Control Policy." Washington: National Academy of Sciences.

Moore, Mark H. 1973. "Policies to Achieve Discrimination on the Effective Price of Heroin." *American Economic Review* 63: 270–277.

———. 1977. *Buy and Bust: The Effective Regulation of an Illicit Market for Heroin.* Lexington, Mass.: Lexington Books.

———. 1990. "Supply Reduction and Drug Law Enforcement." In Michael Tonry and James Q. Wilson, eds., *Drugs and Crime: Crime and Justice,* vol. 13. Chicago: University of Chicago Press.

Moore, Mark H., and Dean R. Gerstein, eds. 1981. *Alcohol and Public Policy: Beyond the Shadow of Prohibition.* Washington: National Academy of Sciences Press.

Musto, David. 1973. *The American Disease*. New Haven: Yale University Press.

National Commission on Marihuana and Drug Abuse. 1973. "Drug Use in America: Problem in Perspective." Washington: Government Printing Office.

Office of National Drug Control Policy. 1999a. "National Drug Control Strategy." Washington.

———. 1999b. "National Drug Control Strategy: Budget Summary." Washington.

Polich, J. Michael, et al. 1984. "Strategies for Controlling Adolescent Drug Use." Santa Monica: Rand.

Resnik, Hank. n.d. "Youth and Drugs: Society's Mixed Messages." Rockville, Md.: Department of Health and Human Services, Public Health Service, Alcohol, Drug Abuse, and Mental Health Administration.

Reuter, Peter, and Mark Kleiman. 1986. "Risks and Prices: An Economic Analysis of Drug Enforcement." In Michael Tonry, ed., *Crime and Justice: An Annual Review of Research,* vol. 7. Chicago: University of Chicago Press.

Reuter, Peter, Gordon Crawford, and Jonathan Cave. 1988. "Sealing the Borders: The Effects of Increased Military Participation in Drug Interdiction." Santa Monica: Rand.

Reuter, Peter, Robert MacCoun, and Patrick Murphy. 1990. *Money from Crime: A Study of the Economics of Drug Dealing in Washington, D.C.* Santa Monica: Rand.

Rydell, C. Peter, and Susan S. Everingham. 1994. "Controlling Cocaine: Supply v. Demand Programs." Santa Monica: Rand.

Sviridoff, Michele, et al. 1992. "Neighborhood Effects of Street-Level Drug Enforcement: An Evaluation of Tactical Narcotics Teams by the Vera Institute of Justice." New York: Vera Institute.

Tragler, Gernot, Jonathan P. Caulkins, and Gustav Feichtinger. 1997. "Optimal Dynamic Allocation of Treatment and Enforcement in Illicit Drug Control." Vienna University of Technology.

Drug Users and Drug Dealers

William N. Brownsberger

Who uses drugs? Who deals drugs? Where do they live? Are they otherwise criminals? These questions are crucial to understanding the mechanics, merits, and politics of alternative approaches to drug control. In this chapter I offer an overview of the available evidence.

Drug Use

Experimentation with illegal drugs has been widespread in the United States. According to the National Household Survey on Drug Abuse, over one-third of Americans have tried an illegal drug (SAMHSA 1999b, table 3B). Prevalence of drug use varies over time. Among those who were young in the early 1980s, few completely avoided illegal drugs: 81 percent of those who graduated from high school in 1981 and 1982 had tried an illegal drug by 1995 when they were 31 or 32; 60 percent had tried an illegal drug other than marijuana; and 37 percent had tried cocaine.[1]

Adolescents and young adults are much more likely than older adults to begin using drugs. Few initiate drug use after the age of 30. The strength of this generalization varies over time. Drug initiation by older adults was relatively high during the explosion of drug use in the late 1960s and early 1970s, although still far lower than drug initiation by the young.[2] In the mid-1990s marijuana and cocaine initiation rates for those aged 12–17 were at historic highs, while initiations for those over 26 were a fraction of their previous peaks. Despite these variations, from the 1960s into the 1990s the average ages of new users of marijuana and cocaine remained in the teens or early twenties, with new cocaine users generally three or four years older than new marijuana users (SAMHSA 1999b, tables 41–42).

The most recent wave of drug use expanded from the late 1960s to a peak around 1980, with marijuana peaking before cocaine. Use of illegal drugs in all age groups trended sharply downward during the 1980s. In the early 1990s drug use was stable among those over 25 but began to trend back up among youths. Between 1992 and 1997 admitted past-month marijuana use among high school seniors doubled from 11.9 to 23.7 percent—but this was still below past-month use by the peak-user class of 1978 (37.1 percent).[3] In 1997 past-month heroin use, although rare among seniors at 0.5 percent, was near its highest level since the beginning of the seniors survey in 1975.[4]

The 1980s fall in drug use correlated with a rise in disapproval and perceived dangerousness of drug use, and the 1990s upturn correlated with a softening of attitudes (NIDA 1999, ch. 8). The upturn sparked heated debate at the national level and led at mid-decade to a resurgence of broad governmental efforts to influence attitudes toward drugs.[5] In the late 1990s drug use among youth generally appeared to level off, with trends slightly varying by drug; perceived dangerousness of drug use also leveled off, but it is too soon to be confident about the longer-term direction of young people's drug use (Johnston, O'Malley, and Bachman 1999, tables 4 and 9; SAMHSA 1999b, ch. 2).

In every age group admitted lifetime experience with illegal drugs among (non-Hispanic) whites is as common or more common than among (non-Hispanic) blacks or Hispanics.[6] Current use—use in the past month—is roughly equally distributed across racial/ethnic groups (see Table 2.1). Apart from the maturation patterns by age (which are similar for all groups), the most striking fact in Table 2.1 is that whites much more frequently admit past-month use of alcohol. All other racial/ethnic differences in the table are small in absolute magnitude and many are not statistically significant. Small but statistically significant differences include lower rates of current illegal drug use

Table 2.1 Current drug experience—used in the past month? (Answers by age bracket from 1998 survey)

	Whites				Blacks				Hispanics			
	12–17	18–25	26–34	35+	12–17	18–25	26–34	35+	12–17	18–25	26–34	35+
Any illicit drug	10.3	17.6	7.1	3.2	9.9	17.1	9.4	4.8	9.9	11.1	5.4	3.5
Marijuana	8.7	14.9	5.7	2.5	8.3	15.2	7.4	3.3	7.6	9.0	3.2	2.4
Cocaine	0.9	2.2	1.0	0.3	*	0.6	2.7	1.3	1.4	2.7	1.1	0.9
Crack	0.3	0.4	0.2	*	*	0.2	1.4	1.1	0.5	0.3	0.1	0.2
Hallucinogens	2.3	3.5	0.3	0.2	0.5	0.3	*	0.1	0.9	1.9	1.1	0.1
Heroin	*	*	*	*	*	*	*	*	*	*	*	*
Alcohol	20.9	65.0	65.2	56.2	13.1	50.3	54.8	38.3	18.9	50.8	53.1	47.7

* Indicates low precision; no estimate reported. Thirty-day heroin estimates by age and race are not provided in the household survey.
Source: SAMHSA 1999a (compilation from tables). Monthly heroin use is too rare to measure in the survey population. Statements of statistical significance in the text are based on the nonoverlap of 95% confidence intervals provided in the source tables.

among Hispanics in the college age bracket, 18–25; higher rates of hallucinogen use among young whites; and higher rates of cocaine and crack use among older blacks.

Studies analyzing smaller subpopulations reveal additional modest variations.[7] Also, group patterns of drug use vary over time. Before the 1960s, lifetime experience with cocaine and marijuana use was more common among blacks than among whites. The crossover occurred in the baby-boom generation.[8]

National survey data show a modest contrast in use prevalence across socioeconomic levels. In the 1997 National Household Survey, for example, those with incomes below $9,000 were almost twice as likely to be past-year users of cocaine and marijuana as those with incomes over $40,000. There were similar 2-to-1 contrasts between those without and those with health insurance and between those collecting and those not collecting welfare. It is worth noting that these socioeconomic contrasts were weaker or nonexistent at the high school (12–17) and college (18–25) ages (SAMHSA 1999d, tables 13.1 and 13.2). The contrasts are equally consistent with the view that frequent drug use may damage one's career and with the view that poverty and instability contribute to frequent drug use. The overall gradient of use prevalence across income levels is modest enough that the vast majority of those with recent drug use experience are not poor.[9]

Self-reports of stigmatized behavior are inherently unreliable. The accuracy of self-reports may vary across groups. Less advantaged groups are harder to locate and interview in household settings. But the basic findings of the national surveys are unquestioned among experts. Lifetime drug use experience is widespread across demographic and socioeconomic groups, including middle-income non-Hispanic whites. The official summary of these findings is: "[D]rugs are not a problem just for inner-city residents, or the poor, or members of some minority group—they affect all Americans from every social, ethnic, racial and economic background" (ONDCP 1996).

The strongest predictors of recent illicit drug use are age and gender (not race or socioeconomic status).[10] Overall, males account for roughly two-thirds (62.4 percent) of past-month illicit drug users (13,615,000 in 1998). Similarly, young (12–34) persons of both gen-

ders account for roughly two-thirds (67.6 percent) of past-month illicit drug users (SAMHSA 1999a, table 2A). It is fair to think of the
"typical" past-month drug user as a young male, probably white
(three out of four). Two-thirds of these typical drug users also drink
heavily or in binges. Of these drinking drug users, almost half smoke
marijuana very heavily—three or more times weekly.[11]

Heavy Drug Use

As clearly as the national surveys show that drug use is widely distributed across all groups in our society, other data show that frequent
cocaine use and frequent heroin use are far more prevalent in urban
poverty populations than elsewhere.[12]

Surveys are limited in three ways in their ability to measure cocaine
and heroin use. First, since cocaine use and heroin use are particularly
stigmatized behaviors, respondents are especially likely to deny them.
Second, since frequent cocaine use and frequent heroin use are often
associated with residential instability, many frequent users may be
hard to locate in a household survey. Third, since frequent cocaine use
and frequent heroin use are relatively rare, general population samples
lack statistical power to accurately measure their contours. While in
the general population reached by the National Household Survey in
1998 only 0.3 percent (roughly 100 actual interviewees) used cocaine
weekly or more often (SAMHSA 1999a, table 21A), interviews of frequent cocaine users indicate that many use cocaine every day ten or
more times per day (e.g. Edlin et al. 1994). The total amount of cocaine estimated to be consumed in the United States based on responses to the National Household Survey is an order of magnitude
less than the amount estimated to be consumed based on production
and seizure estimates.[13]

Frequent cocaine and heroin users become accessible to measurement through their contacts with the health care and criminal justice
systems. Over the past decade the use of drug testing in these systems
has led to an understanding that a large population of frequent drug
users is invisible to the National Household Survey and that these frequent users reside disproportionately in urban poverty areas.

Drug Testing of Arrestees

The federal government's Drug Use Forecasting system provided the first indication of widespread drug use undetected by survey instruments. DUF, recently expanded and renamed ADAM (Arrestee Drug Abuse Monitoring Program), samples adult felony arrestees in 35 cities (National Institute of Justice 1999a). The program administers urine tests to the arrestees and also interviews them. The program grew out of pilot studies in Manhattan and Washington, D.C., in the mid-1980s (Reardon 1993). It has now shown that in most major cities well over half of arrestees test positive for some illegal drug. In 11 of the 35 cities in 1998, the most common illegal drug identified among males was not marijuana but cocaine. Cocaine was most common among females in 28 of the cities (National Institute of Justice 1999b, 4).

The DUF findings for cocaine prevalence had dramatic implications. Cocaine metabolites become undetectable after approximately 72 hours. The finding that many arrestees tested positive for cocaine indicated that many of them must be frequent cocaine users. As the DUF program found high cocaine prevalence in more and more cities, analysts realized that there must be a great many more frequent cocaine users than the Household Survey estimated. They also realized that many of the frequent cocaine users must have been arrested at least once in the past year, although not necessarily for a drug offense.

Questions about prior arrests added to the National Household Survey suggest that the survey is ineffective in reaching (and/or getting candid answers from) the arrestee population: the survey data suggest a total of 5.9 million arrests in 1997, while the FBI estimates 15.3 million.[14] Equally discrepant, the survey data suggest that among male past-year arrestees in 1997, only 4.7 percent were weekly or more frequent cocaine users, while in the median ADAM city, 37 percent of male arrestees tested positive for cocaine use in the past three days.[15]

Careful studies of the DUF results addressed a number of factors that might confound interpretation of the test results (e.g. Rhodes 1993; Rhodes et al. 1997). Some frequent cocaine users may not be arrested in a given year. Some may be arrested more than once. Some who test positive for cocaine on arrest may not be frequent users. The large DUF cities may not accurately represent all smaller cities. The offense mixes for offenders selected into the DUF samples vary across DUF sites and so sites are not necessarily comparable or representative. Some of those arrested may also be represented in the survey population. It is now generally accepted that the national surveys radically undercount frequent cocaine users and that a sizeable fraction of frequent cocaine users are arrested at least once every year (Rhodes et al. 1997, 10, 13; ONDCP 1999, 13; ONDCP 1998, 7).

The size of the hidden population of frequent cocaine users is subject to considerable uncertainty, despite the careful estimating work done to date. The Household Survey estimates 600,000 frequent (weekly or more often) cocaine users in 1998, and this figure has changed little since the mid-1980s (see SAMHSA 1999b, 36). SAMHSA researchers estimate that the actual figure may be 20–40 percent higher than their survey indicates (ibid., 43). The Office of National Drug Control Policy quoted a figure 500 percent higher— 3.6 million frequent cocaine users—in its 1998 and 1999 strategies, but used a figure of 2.1 million in its 1994 strategy. Both ONDCP estimates are from similar models using the DUF data but with a key estimating parameter changed—the frequency of arrests of cocaine users.[16] The more often users are arrested, the fewer there need be to account for the known number of arrestees who test positive for cocaine. The Office of National Drug Control Policy has recognized the uncertainty and has funded pilot work toward more reliable estimates (Simeone et al. 1997; ONDCP 1998, 6).

Given that some large portion of frequent cocaine users are not reflected in the Household Survey, it follows that the survey findings of a broad distribution of drug abuse across society do not necessarily apply to frequent cocaine use. We must look to other indicators to understand the epidemiology of frequent cocaine use. The finding that arrestees account for a large share of the cocaine users has distributional implications when combined with data about the distribution of arrests. An extensive literature recognizes that crime and arrests are several times more prevalent in poverty areas (see Brownsberger 1997a, 1997b). It appears then that frequent cocaine use is also several times more prevalent in poverty areas.

Frequent cocaine abusers in nonpoverty areas may be less frequently incarcerated, either because they are under less economic
pressure to commit crimes or because law enforcement treats them
differently. If hard-to-measure neighborhood and racial variation in
the arrest rates for frequent cocaine users were wide enough to offset
the measured differences in neighborhood arrest rates, then the infer-
ence of wide prevalence contrasts could be questioned. Other indicators tend to negate this possibility.

Other Indicators of Frequent Use

Many hospitals have conducted studies of newborns and mothers in
their hospitals to measure the prevalence of cocaine exposure among
newborns. These studies generally test large random samples—they do
not target mothers or babies with particular risk factors. Tests in some
suburban hospitals serving relatively affluent clienteles reveal exposure rates under 1 percent. In some urban hospitals serving poverty
populations, tests reveal exposure rates over 30 percent. When the results from this corpus of studies are arrayed, the higher prevalence of
exposure in poverty areas is strongly indicated (Brownsberger 1997a).

Data on treatment admissions also tend to support a finding of a
strong differential in frequent cocaine abuse across neighborhood
poverty levels. Treatment admissions are, of course, a function not
only of use levels but also of treatment seeking. And available data
about treatment admissions omit some private facilities. But the available data suggest a strong differential in need for treatment across income levels. Treatment admissions for cocaine and heroin are 18
times more prevalent in the poorest 10 percent of zip codes in Massachusetts than in the wealthiest. The poorest 10 percent of the state accounts for 32 percent of the state's treatment admissions (Brownsberger 1997b).

The Drug Abuse Warning Network tracks mentions of drug abuse
in emergency room admissions. The hospitals sampled are designed to
represent hospitals in the country as a whole. Two observations from
this data set support the notion of a hidden population of cocaine
abusers concentrated in poverty areas. First, two-thirds of all of the
emergency room mentions of cocaine use pertain to blacks and Hispanics, who are relatively highly concentrated in poverty areas.[17] Sec-

ond, while frequent cocaine use measured by the Household Survey has been level since the mid-1980s and overall use has fallen, emergency room mentions of cocaine have increased dramatically. They grew fourfold from 1985 to 1989, then increased approximately 55 percent from 1989 to 1998.[18] While there is some evidence of increased mentions among those under 17, most of the recent growth in mentions has been among those over 35, consistent with the possibility that an aging group of cocaine users is experiencing increasing medical difficulties.[19]

Survey studies concentrating on poverty areas or on the homeless also reveal a radically higher prevalence of cocaine use than in the general population. Similarly, ethnographic studies of urban poverty populations include extensive impressions of frequent cocaine use. While there is a literature dating to the early 1980s portraying cocaine abuse in elite circles, there is little to suggest widespread frequent cocaine abuse in Middle America in the 1990s (Brownsberger 1997a).

Summary of Evidence on Cocaine Use

While cocaine once was seen as a glamorous drug, the available evidence indicates that frequent cocaine use is now far more prevalent in urban poverty areas than elsewhere. Frequent cocaine users are often homeless (Simeone et al. 1997) and frequently arrested. At this point they are, in many regions, an aging group. Many of the frequent users appear to have acquired their habits during the early stages of the epidemic.

There is a good deal that the evidence leaves unclear. First, although it is generally agreed that frequent users account for the bulk of cocaine and heroin consumption (e.g. Rhodes et al. 1997; Everingham and Rydell 1994), we know little about the distribution of consumption levels within the "frequent" user category. Consumption is impossible to measure for the disorganized crack user; estimates derived from self-reports vary widely, but in some instances exceed one gram per day (e.g. Ratner 1992; Washton 1987). On the other hand, one estimate of average consumption among frequent users places it at 0.2 grams per day.[20] This suggests the possibility of considerable variation in use levels among "frequent" cocaine users. It is also consistent with the notion that cocaine users binge episodically. We could speculate that younger more successful hustler-addicts typically spend heavily while burnt-out partially disabled addicts may scrape by on limited cocaine doses. Many other scenarios are possible.

Second, we do not know how many of the frequent users would meet criteria for addiction. Use levels in themselves do not define addiction. Measures of addiction turn on dependence, on subjective experiences of loss of control over use, and on negative consequences of drug use. Given the abject conditions of many frequent cocaine users, one might infer widespread clinical addiction in the group, but it is also possible that in some instances abject conditions may have preceded frequent use and the frequent use may not rise to the level of addiction.

Third, we do not know the turnover rates of the frequent user population. Do the frequent users cycle out of frequent use, or is there a stable population stuck at high use levels? The sketchy evidence suggests a fairly stable population. Lower rates of use among younger arrestees suggest that the inflow to the frequent user population may have dropped (although recent rate increases among young arrestees in some cities raise concern; National Institute of Justice 1999a, 2; 1999b, 11–15). High relapse rates and data on the length of cocaine-using careers suggest that outflow from the frequent user population is slow.

Fourth, while we know that frequent cocaine use is much more prevalent in urban poverty areas, we do not know what overall proportion of the universe of frequent users is concentrated in those areas. The measurement frameworks for our various kinds of data associating use prevalence with poverty rates are incommensurate. We cannot associate levels of use prevalence with specific poverty rates. And, in the few instances where we have good local statistics, we cannot safely generalize to national statistics.

Frequent Use of Drugs Other Than Cocaine

The profile of frequent heroin users resembles the profile of frequent cocaine users—socioeconomically disadvantaged. The same basic argument for high concentration of cocaine use in poverty areas (most users are arrested and arrestees are concentrated in poverty areas) applies to heroin. Frequent cocaine use remains far more prevalent than frequent heroin use.

In the early 1990s increased availability of cheap, pure heroin in many cities and increases in some indicators of heroin use led to fears of a broad new epidemic of heroin addiction (e.g. Drug Enforcement Administration 1996). At the close of the decade, from a national perspective, it appeared that the worst fears had not so far been realized. Perceived heroin availability jumped in the late 1980s but was roughly level throughout the 1990s.[21] Initiations of heroin use as reflected in the Household Survey increased in the early 1990s, but did not increase from 1994 to 1997, and heroin initiations are still only a fraction of cocaine initiations.[22] Reported heroin use prevalence also appears to have stabilized in the late 1990s at a level well below reported cocaine use prevalence, even among youths.[23] Similarly, emergency room mentions of heroin increased in the early 1990s, but appear to have been stable since 1995, again at a level considerably below cocaine mentions.[24] Heroin treatment admissions rose in the early 1990s but have been roughly level since 1994 (SAMHSA 1999g, table 2.1). The early 1990s increases in emergency room heroin mentions and heroin treatment admissions were both driven primarily by increases among older users, as opposed to new young users.[25]

The data from drug testing of arrestees support a computation that heavy heroin use is more prevalent than the surveys indicate. But even in this computation heavy heroin use is still considerably rarer than heavy cocaine use.[26] Further, the drug testing data do not support a finding of a general increase in heavy heroin use, with fewer arrestees testing positive for heroin in 1998 than in 1990 in many major cities.[27] Heroin positive tests remained essentially constant around 8 percent of arrestees from 1990 to 1998 (on average across widely varying ADAM cities), and cocaine positive tests remained approximately five times as common as heroin positive tests.[28] It may be that early 1990s heroin increases were concentrated among older long-term polydrug users who are suffering significant health consequences (reflected in the emergency room and treatment data discussed above), but are beyond their high arrest-rate years.[29] Only 16.1 percent of persons over 18 admitted for heroin treatment in 1997 were employed full-time, and 24.9 percent were homeless (SAMHSA 1999g, tables 3.5 and 3.7).

Cocaine and heroin together account for an estimated 83.7 percent of the nation's expenditures on illegal drugs (Rhodes et al. 1997) and 57.6 percent of treatment admissions excluding alcohol primary admissions (my computation based on SAMHSA 1999g, table 2.1). Marijuana accounts for most of the rest: 12.3 percent of expenditures and 25.1 percent of treatment admissions. Frequent (more than weekly) marijuana use is harder to distinguish through drug testing, because marijuana remains detectable for as long as 30 days after use. The positive marijuana test rates in the ADAM program, of 50.8 percent for males and 35.0 percent for females aged 21–25 in 1998, suggest past-month use prevalence at those levels among arrestees.[30] Those monthly use levels are well above levels measured by the Household Survey for the 18–25 age range—17.2 percent for males and 10.9 percent for females (SAMHSA 1999a, table 3A)—but they give little insight into daily use levels. The implications of the ADAM drug testing data as to the prevalence of marijuana use have received little attention; analysts have been content to rely on the Household Survey (e.g. Rhodes et al. 1997). The ADAM data suggest that, as for cocaine and heroin, there is a subpopulation of criminal marijuana users not well captured in the Household Survey.[31] In the ADAM sample, black, white, and Hispanic positive drug test rates for marijuana are similar.[32] Nationwide, two-thirds of arrestees are whites, usually young males. Whites account for 47.3 percent of marijuana emergency room mentions and 60.2 percent of marijuana treatment admissions (SAMHSA 1999f, table 25; 1999g, table 3.1a). The possible upward adjustment of our estimate of frequent marijuana users may not change our picture of the typical current marijuana user as a young white male, but it does imply a greater overlap between marijuana users and persons with criminal justice system involvement (and probable lower socioeconomic status) than appears in the Household Survey data.

Heavy Alcohol Use

Because alcohol use is so much more widespread and because it is a less stigmatized behavior, the National Household Survey provides a more reasonable estimation of the distribution of heavy alcohol use. The Survey defines heavy alcohol use as five or more drinks on more than five occasions within the past month. Heavy alcohol use (ironically, like abstinence) is slightly more prevalent among persons with lower income and education (Flewelling et al. 1992, tables 3.1 and 3.4). Male gender is the overwhelming predictor of heavy alcohol consumption (ibid., table 5.1), much stronger than age and all other personal characteristics.

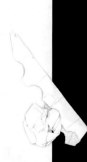

Dealers

Most of our understanding of the demographics of drug-dealing comes from study of the population arrested and charged with drug offenses. Given the difficulties of observing drug dealing, there are no useful statistics related to unarrested drug dealers.

Drug Dealing as Reflected through Law Enforcement

National statistical information shows that blacks and Hispanics are disproportionately represented among those incarcerated for drug dealing. Table 2.2 summarizes statistics from national surveys of criminal justice populations. It shows, for example, that blacks represent 56 percent of all state drug prisoners nationwide. Most of those imprisoned for drug offenses were convicted of trafficking as opposed to possession.[33]

Incarcerations for drug offenses are a major component of high state and federal incarceration rates for blacks and Hispanics. Among black state prisoners, as the table shows, 25 percent are drug prisoners. Seven percent of black males in their twenties and thirties were sentenced prisoners in 1997 (Bureau of Justice Statistics 1999a, 10). Overall prison incarceration rates for blacks were roughly 2.5 times higher than for Hispanics and 8 times higher than for whites (ibid., table 15). In addition to the over one million prisoners sentenced for one year or more, there are another half million persons awaiting trial or sentenced to terms under one year, and another almost 4 million persons on probation or parole (Bureau of Justice Statistics 1999b, table 1.1). It appears that current criminal justice supervision rates for young black males may exceed 30 percent nationwide.[34]

Table 2.2

Sentenced prisoners (one year or more)	Total prisoners	Drug as % of total	Drug offenders as % of group			Group as % of drug offenders		
			Black	Hispanic	White	Black	Hispanic	White
Sentenced state prisoners, 1997[a]	1,100,500	21	25	27	12	56	23	19
Growth in sentenced state prisoners 1990–1997[b]	410,900	19	24	18	11	62	16	18
Sentenced federal prisoners, 1998[c]	95,552	59			N/A[d]			
Growth in sentenced federal prisoners, 1990–1998[e]	47,675	66						

a. Computations based on Bureau of Justice Statistics 1999a, table 16.
b. Computations based on Bureau of Justice Statistics 1999a, tables 17–18.
c. May 1998 data from the Federal Bureau of Prisons online at www.bop.gov, accessed Dec. 31, 1999.
d. The sources referred to in notes a–c do not provide population counts for 1998 by race. According to data from the Federal Bureau of Prisons, Office of Research and Evaluation, Statistical Reporting Section, the number of federal drug prisoners in Sept. 1998 was 55,638; they were 44.6% black and 31.6% Hispanic, but these are overlapping categories—53.9% were classified as white.
e. Sept. 1990 and May 1998 data from the Federal Bureau of Prisons online at www.bop.gov, accessed Dec. 31, 1999.

While these incarceration and supervision rates are high, and growth in drug incarcerations has made a significant contribution to them, it appears that drug incarcerations may have leveled off in the late 1990s. After 478 percent growth from 1985 to 1995, the estimated number of state drug prisoners held steady from 1995 to 1996 and actually dropped slightly from 1996 to 1997, while prisoners serving time for violent or public order offenses continued to grow (Bureau of Justice Statistics 1997, table 13; 1998, table 15; 1999a, table 16). At the federal level the drug prisoner count continued to rise, but more slowly than the nondrug prisoner count.[35]

National data do not measure the neighborhood distribution of prosecutions for drug trafficking. My study of the state prison population in Massachusetts (Brownsberger 1997b) provided the first quantification of the very powerful association between neighborhood poverty levels and incarceration for drug-dealing offenses. The study focused on state as opposed to minor county incarcerations. At the state level in Massachusetts, 99.2 percent of drug prisoners were convicted of dealing offenses and 99.7 percent were convicted of offenses involving cocaine or heroin. In Massachusetts the poorest 10 percent of neighborhoods have drug incarceration rates 56 times higher than the wealthiest 10 percent of neighborhoods. The wealthier 50 percent of the neighborhoods account for only 8.9 percent of drug incarcerations. The study showed that dealing incarceration rates are strongly and independently influenced both by neighborhood poverty and by race/ethnicity but that the race/ethnicity differences are strongest—the Hispanic rate of incarceration for dealing is 83 times greater than the white rate (ibid., charts 12–13 and tables 36–37).

Interpreting the Law Enforcement Data

Of course, the results of the law enforcement process reflect a host of factors other than the underlying prevalence of drug dealing. First, it is possible that poverty forces easy-to-detect street dealing, while wealth allows discreet indoor transactions. Yet, while destructive open-air markets are largely confined to poverty areas, dealing in poverty areas also occurs indoors in crack houses and housing projects. The phenomenon of open-air markets highlights the prevalence of dealing in many poverty areas. It does not indicate a lack of hidden indoor dealing in poverty areas.

Second, although studies have concluded that any racial bias has only a modest effect on overall arrest rates (see Tonry 1995), blacks and Hispanics may be more likely to be stopped, searched, and charged with drug possession. However, this reality is unlikely to affect dealing arrest rates significantly. To make a dealing case, an undercover officer must usually complete a hand-to-hand transaction with the dealer. Anecdotal evidence indicates that white narcotics officers are not very effective in targeting black and Hispanic drug dealers. White undercover officers often prefer to infiltrate white organizations where they share more background with the targets and can be more effective. As one works higher in the drug distribution chain, the relationship that the undercover officer must attain becomes more intimate and the disadvantage of white officers in targeting minorities becomes greater. Over 80 percent of law enforcement officers nationwide are white non-Hispanics (Maguire and Pastore 1997, tables 1.15, 1.32, 1.33).

Third, political leaders may commit more police resources to urban poverty areas with high minority populations—an aggregate version of the previous concern. I am unaware of any studies comparing the neighborhood-level deployment of police officers with poverty rates within cities. However, cities in the aggregate have more police officers per capita than suburban areas. But on a per crime basis, cities often have fewer officers. Urban police officers have to spend proportionately more of their time addressing serious violent crime.[36] Consistent with this statistical fact, anecdotal evidence indicates that the resources committed to known drug problems are, in many instances, greater in non-poverty areas. In general, there is every reason to believe that poverty areas need more police attention rather than less (see Walinsky 1995).

Fourth, as to post-arrest outcomes, lack of high-quality representation and racial discrimination introduce bias into prosecution decisions, pretrial and trial processes, and sentencing. While these phenomena are indisputable, few analysts now believe that they introduce distortion great enough to account for a sizeable portion of the disproportionality in drug incarceration rates (Tonry 1995; see also Brownsberger 1997b).

At the highest levels Colombians and Mexicans dominate the cocaine market. They also control much of the high-level marijuana and heroin trade. It is unsurprising that Hispanics are disproportionately represented in high-level drug-trafficking convictions. Since blacks and Hispanics often reside in close proximity in poverty areas, it is unsurprising that blacks are also disproportionately represented among dealers.

As a last check on the conclusion that poverty areas are the primary (but not exclusive) location for drug trafficking, consider the anecdotal evidence about the flow of buyers from place to place. One rarely hears of inner-city youths traveling as buyers to the suburbs. By contrast, it is a law enforcement commonplace that suburban drug users come to the city to buy from urban dealers. It is also a commonplace that suburban dealers buy drugs in quantity from city wholesalers.

Much of the criminal justice system data supporting a finding that blacks and Hispanics in poverty areas have a lead role in the drug trade applies to cocaine and heroin but not to marijuana. FBI arrest data show that while 57.6 percent of adults arrested for selling cocaine or heroin are black, only 35.0 percent of adults arrested for selling marijuana are black. Only 27.6 percent of adults arrested for possessing marijuana are black.[37] Perhaps for the very reason that so many white middle-class youths use and sell marijuana, sentencing policies for marijuana possession and trafficking are lighter than for cocaine and heroin. As a result, the heavy representation of blacks and Hispanics and residents of urban poverty areas among the population incarcerated for drug-trafficking offenses reflects primarily their leadership in the cocaine and heroin trade. The marijuana trade may be considerably less concentrated among minorities and in poverty areas.

Relationship to Crime and Violence

Are Drug Users Otherwise Criminals?

Drug use and alcohol use are associated with criminal offending. Two facts are known with certainty. First, daily use of cocaine or heroin often causes high rates of income-producing crime—robbery, burglary, theft, prostitution, and drug dealing. Addicts are at once impaired as lawful workers and in need of a high income stream to support their habit. Interview studies of prisoners and treatment clients have shown that their frequency of criminal offending is significantly correlated with their rates of hard-drug consumption (Chaiken and Chaiken 1990). Second, heavy substance abuse often leads to destructive behavior. This behavior may be illegal or merely wrong. Marriages and careers may deteriorate. The user may be cruel to or withdraw from family members and friends. The user may drive while intoxicated. The user may misbehave publicly or become involved in violence, ending up injured or injuring others.[38]

What is not so clearly known is how lighter substance use affects criminality. For an unemployed and homeless user, even a very modest habit may create pressure to commit income-producing crimes. However, cross-sectional and longitudinal studies both suggest that the causal links between light drug use and criminality are weak. First, the numbers of those using substances casually greatly exceeds the number of persons arrested every year.[39] Second, longitudinal study of youths shows that delinquency precedes drug use more often than the reverse. Longitudinal study also shows that while delinquency usually ends with adulthood, drug use often continues into adulthood. "Use of illicit drugs does not appear to be strongly related to onset and participation in predatory crime; rather, drug use and crime participation are weakly related as contemporaneous products of factors generally antithetical to traditional United States lifestyles" (Chaiken and Chaiken 1990, 234). Of course, substance abuse may directly cause crimes like disorderly conduct or driving while intoxicated.

The link between *non-income-producing* violent crime and drug use is not well established. Some types of intoxication may in some settings make some users more likely to commit violent crime, but for other individuals or other drugs or other settings the effect may be the opposite. The statistical role of addiction and intoxication in the causation of non-income-producing violent crime is a question likely to remain unsettled (Fagan 1990). Professionals in the criminal justice system believe on the basis of their own observations that many offenders abuse substances (e.g. see Massachusetts Supreme Judicial Court 1995). The ADAM data from drug testing of arrested persons confirm that use is widespread among offenders. For many, it seems counterintuitive that illegal drug use is often not a cause but merely a correlate of crime.

Dealers and Violence

Many drug dealers are dangerous violent criminals. Some observers have suggested that a capacity for explosive violence is a prerequisite to success in the business. There are no legal methods to enforce contracts, thus only violence or the threat of violence can help to resolve disputes. Some dealers at a higher level regularly conduct transactions in which large sums of money are exchanged for drugs. The risk of robbery in any one of these transactions is great. Higher-level dealers may extend credit to subordinate dealers and need to collect from them. They may police a large turf belonging to them. This image of the drug dealer as a particularly dangerous criminal has wide currency in the public mind. It motivates harsh sentencing policies. Undoubtedly, there are many dealers that fit this profile.

The reality may be more complex. Studies of the criminal records of drug traffickers show that many of them have previously been charged with violent offenses, but that many others have not (e.g. Brownsberger 1997b). There is considerable diversity in the roles of dealers. It is plausible that success at a higher level often does require a capacity for violence, but that low-level retail dealers may not need the same skills. They are not trusted with large quantities of cash or drugs. They do not extend credit, but only do cash-on-delivery transactions. They may function under the turf-protection umbrella of their supplier. They may be frequent victims of low-level robbers and of disciplinary violence from their suppliers, but cope primarily through avoidance and compliance. They may be users themselves. They may deal on only a part-time basis as a modest supplement to a day job.

There is no good reason to believe that any generalization about violence or lack thereof among lower-level dealers should hold across all areas. It may be that in some markets the drug trade is entirely dominated by violent gangs, organized all the way down to the retail level. In other areas, relatively nonviolent dealers under the disciplinary control of violent gang members may conduct the retail trade. In some areas, turf may not be clearly allocated and some nonviolent user-dealers may deal casually.

In Washington, D.C., Peter Reuter and his colleagues have shown that roughly 30 percent of the young black men were arrested for drug dealing between 1985 and 1991 (Saner, MacCoun, and Reuter 1996). More were arrested for drug dealing than for all nondrug felonies combined. An interview study of a sample of arrested dealers (Reuter et al. 1990) found that 64 percent held legitimate jobs and moonlighted part-time as dealers. Their net earnings from drug dealing of $30 per hour dramatically exceeded their typical legitimate wage of roughly $7 per hour. Most of them earned more from their moonlighting than from their full-time work. Most earned little or nothing from other types of crime. Only 27 percent had ever been arrested for a violent crime. Over half used drugs themselves. Washington in the late 1980s may have been a market that included some relatively nonviolent casual user-dealers.

Summary

The main conclusions from this tour of the demographics of drug use and drug dealing are as follows:

- Drug users come from all racial/ethnic groups and all socioeconomic strata.
- Heavy users of cocaine or heroin reside disproportionately in poverty areas.
- Heavy use of cocaine or heroin tends to result in high rates of crime, and heavy users of cocaine or heroin are arrested quite frequently.
- Moderate drug use may or may not increase the probability of criminal offending, although there is a clear ecological association between drug use and crime.
- Drug dealers and those incarcerated for drug-dealing offenses reside disproportionately in poverty areas and are disproportionately black and Hispanic.
- Some drug dealers are violent; others injure society mainly by selling drugs.

It should be recognized that these facts are contemporary contingent realities. For example, cocaine abuse might have waxed and waned as a primarily middle-class epidemic in the 1980s if crack had never been developed. Crack facilitated the marketing of cocaine in small doses and fueled the explosion of cocaine abuse and related violence in poverty areas in the late 1980s. As middle-class demand fell, prices dropped even in the face of efforts to control supply. The most recent evidence offers some modest encouragement, but communities differ widely and many will see their problems worsen before they improve.

Notes

This chapter was produced with the generous support of the Harpel foundation.

1. Data from the Monitoring the Future survey (NIDA 1997, 37).
2. The youth and early adulthood of most of those over 50 in 1996 predated the explosion of drug use in the late 1960s. In 1996, among those aged 35–49 who had tried marijuana, 98.3 percent had tried it before age 30. But among those over 50 who had tried marijuana, only 64.5 percent had tried it before age 30. My calculations based on 1996 National Household Survey Data using the online Survey Data Analysis system made available through the Substance Abuse and Mental Health Data Archive at www.icpsr.umich.edu/SAMHDA as released in June 1998 (SAMHSA 1998b). See Harrison et al. 1995 on Gallup polling results showing a jump in lifetime marijuana experience from 5 percent of college students in 1967 to 51 percent in 1971. SAMHSA 1999b, table 41, provides age-specific rates of marijuana initiation, 1965–1997.
3. SAMHSA 1998a, tables 2.6 and 2.7, past-month and past-year use. Johnston, O'Malley, and Bachman 1999. NIDA 1999, table 5–3.
4. It was slightly below its 1995 level of 0.6 percent. Through most of the 1980s and early 1990s it was at 0.2 percent. Johnston, O'Malley, and Bachman 1999.
5. See, e.g., House of Representatives, Committee on Government Reform and Oversight 1995. Compare the Office of National Drug Control Policy's National Drug Control Strategies of 1994 and 1998. The latter puts a much greater emphasis on prevention through attitude leadership.
6. SAMHSA 1999a, tables 2B, 2C, 2D. By "as common or more common" I mean that there is no statistical difference (as for the 12–17 age group) or whites are higher by a statistically significant amount (as for all other age groups).

7. See SAMHSA 1999c for a finer analysis of relative prevalence among racial/ethnic subgroups. This analysis shows, for example, that past-year illicit drug use rates among Puerto Rican Americans and Mexican Americans are roughly twice the rates among some other Hispanic groups, but still less than 1.5 percentage points above the national average rate of 11.9 percent.

8. Inferences from Johnson et al. 1996, which analyzes retrospective data from the 1991–1993 National Household Surveys in which participants were asked when they first used marijuana and cocaine.

9. My analysis of the 1996 National Household Survey Data as in note 3 shows that past-month cocaine and marijuana use prevalence are elevated among those receiving public assistance and those with family incomes below $20,000. However, over 90 percent of past-month users are not on welfare and over 70 percent have family incomes above $20,000.

10. See Flewelling, Rachal, and Marsden 1992, tables 5.3 and 5.5. Among factors predicting past-month marijuana or cocaine use or (age, gender, race, education, occupation, marital status, employment status, number of jobs in past five years, and number of moves in past five years), age and gender are the strongest. The one exception is that divorced or never-married status is a stronger predictor of cocaine use than gender (but not age). See also prevalence cross-tabulations in SAMHSA 1999d.

11. My analysis of the 1997 National Household Survey Data as in note 3. SAMHSA 1999e.

12. The word "frequent" is used most commonly to refer to use weekly or more often, but most of the available data on cocaine and heroin use do not allow good quantification of the frequency of use.

13. Everingham and Rydell multiply per-person consumption estimates and population estimates from the National Household Survey in 1990 to derive an estimated annual consumption of 19.3 metric tons of cocaine. They note that law enforcement agencies seize about 100 tons per year and that it is implausible that the government is seizing the majority of the cocaine entering the country. Moreover, estimates based on coca crop cultivation place total cocaine available for consumption after interdiction at approximately 300 metric tons per year. Rydell and Everingham 1994, table A.8. The Household Survey no longer asks about amount of cocaine consumption.

14. My calculations from the 1997 Household Survey (SAMHSA 1999e) as in note 3. Federal Bureau of Investigation 1999, section 4.

15. My calculations from the 1997 Household Survey (SAMHSA 1999e) as in note 3 and National Institute of Justice 1999a, 3.

16. See ONDCP 1994, 14; 1998, 7; 1999, 13; and compare Rhodes 1993, 306 (.87 arrests per year) with Rhodes et al. 1997, n12 (.5 arrests per year). Rhodes et al. 1997 estimate 3.2 million frequent users in 1990; Rhodes 1993 estimates the 1990 count at 2.1 million. The 1997 estimate

actually uses a more stringent definition of "frequent" or "hardcore"—use on 10 days in the past month as opposed to weekly use—for the portion of the estimate derived from arrestee data. In the 1997 survey data only about 200,000 met the more stringent criterion, while about 600,000 met the weekly use criterion. My calculations from the 1997 Household Survey (SAMHSA 1999e) as in note 3. This makes the upward revision even more striking.

17. Nationwide in 1992 blacks accounted for 47.9 percent of the population residing in central-city poverty areas.

18. My calculation based on SAMHSA 1996, 7, and SAMHSA 1999f, table 21. This is an approximate computation because it is based on first half-year data for 1998.

19. SAMHSA 1999f, table 21. Both the increase in youth emergency room mentions and the dominance of adult mentions are broadly consistent with data from the ADAM system, which show increases in youth use in some cities but show the highest rates among over-30 arrestees in most cities. National Institute of Justice 1999b, 11–12.

20. This follows from Rhodes et al. (1997), who derive average per-user expenditure of $187 per week from the DUF data and prices of $139 per pure gram from DEA reports.

21. The number of high school seniors indicating that it would be "fairly easy" or "very easy" to get heroin if they wanted some rose from 21.0 percent in 1985 to 31.9 percent in 1990. In 1999 it was 32.1 percent. Johnston et al. 1999, tables 10–11. It fluctuated between 32 and 36 percent throughout the 1990s. See also SAMHSA 1999b, tables 49– 50.

22. SAMHSA 1999b, tables 42 and 45 and pp. 24–28. Heroin initiations, 1994–1997, were 85, 88, 149, and 81 (thousands), while cocaine initiations were 542, 655, 670, and 730 (thousands). The annual fluctuations in heroin initiations (e.g. from 149,000 down to 81,000 from 1997 to 1998) are not statistically significant, although the increase from the early 1990s levels is statistically significant.

23. SAMHSA 1999b, table 5A and p. 18. Past-year heroin users in the Household Survey actually dropped significantly from 1997 (597,000) to 1998 (235,000)—below the 1994 level. Past-month users also dropped, although wide fluctuations in this small quantity (130,000 in 1998) are not statistically significant. Cocaine use was an order of magnitude more common in the 1998 survey: 3,811,000 past-year users and 1,750,000 past-month users. Similarly, in the high school students survey, both past-year and past-month heroin use (respectively 1.1 percent and 0.5 percent among seniors) were flat from 1995 to 1999, again, considerably below cocaine use (generally one-fourth as common as cocaine among seniors and half as common as cocaine among eighth graders). Johnston et al. 1999.

24. SAMHSA 1999f, table 23 and p. 17. Heroin mentions have fluctuated insignificantly between 35,000 and 39,000 per half year since 1995. For the past two years cocaine mentions have fluctuated around 80,000 per half year, although they have increased from a level around 60,000 since the early 1990s. SAMHSA 1999f, table 1.

25. Only 2.9 percent of heroin treatment admissions were under 20 in 1997. Growth in admissions under 20 accounted for only 9 percent of the 1992–1997 increase. My computations based on SAMHSA 1999g, tables 2.3 and 3.1a. Similarly, those aged 12–17 amounted to only 1.2 percent of all heroin emergency room mentions in the first half of 1998. My computations based on SAMHSA 1999f, table 23.

26. Rhodes, et al. 1997, 13. ONDCP 1999, 13, using an estimate of 810,000 heavy heroin users and 3.6 million heavy cocaine users.

27. National Institute of Justice 1999c, 24. Twelve of the 23 "veteran" (i.e., history available) ADAM sites show decreases in heroin positive test rates among males from 1990 to 1998 (not all of them statistically significant decreases). Rhodes et al. 1997 also shows stable estimates of heavy heroin use based on arrestee testing data between 1988 and 1995.

28. Between 1990 and 1998 the unweighted average cocaine positive rate across the 23 veteran ADAM cities declined from 42.0 to 35.9, the unweighted average heroin positive rate declined from 8.3 to 7.7, and the ratio of cocaine positives to heroin positives declined from 5.1 to 4.7. My calculations from National Institute of Justice 1999b, table 2; 1999c, table 1.

29. Among heroin treatment admissions in 1997, 27.3 percent also used crack and 11.6 percent (possibly overlapping) used powder cocaine. SAMHSA 1999g, table 3.6.

30. Test results averaged across 23 major cities (without weighting), not necessarily representative of all cities or all arrestees. My calculations based on National Institute of Justice 1999d, table 3.

31. One could, based on the ADAM data, reasonably estimate the number of past-year-arrested past-month marijuana users at anywhere from 5 to 15 million as against a Household Survey estimate of 10.1 million past-month users of which only 3.1 million admit *ever* having been arrested and booked. Positive marijuana test rates vary by city size and region, across age, across gender, and across offense categories in the ADAM data. Except for the gender variations, these variations are generally modest and offsetting in the ADAM universe of cities. The gender contrast is wide and consistent, but the ADAM female percentage of 27.5 approximates the nationwide female share of arrestees, 21 percent in 1996. Self-reported past-month use somewhat *exceeds* positive test rates: 52.6 percent of the whole 1996 ADAM sample either tested positive or admitted past-month use while positive tests were at the 36.9 percent level. To ex-

trapolate nationwide, one needs to adjust for the fact that the ADAM sites are all central cities; roughly following Rhodes 1993, one can use the share that drug arrests constitute of total arrests to deflate the central-city ADAM drug-testing data to a national urban/suburban/rural average. In the large cities, the FBI reports that 14.0 percent of arrests are for drug violations, as against 10.2 percent in the nation as a whole. Multiplying $10.2 \div 14.0 \times 52.6$, one gets 38.3 percent; round this to 40 percent. One can compute an average annual arrest frequency from the ADAM data itself (using the number of arrests in the prior 12 months, excluding the current arrest as uncorrelated and ignoring possible incarcerations). This works out to an average .85 arrests per year per user, remarkably close to Rhodes's .87 figure for cocaine users in his first estimate in 1993. Rounding this figure down to .8 (allowing for a modest impact of incarcerations consistent with Rhodes 1993) we can estimate the past-month marijuana users involved with the criminal justice system as $40\% \div .8 \times 15,168,000$ arrests, or 7.6 million persons. My computations using FBI 1997, National Institute of Justice 1998, and SAMHSA 1998b. On the other hand, an arrest rate of 0.4 per year, equally plausible (see Rhodes et al. 1997), would result in an estimate twice as high with greater implications for the social demographics of marijuana users. I use 1996 data here (National Institute of Justice 1998, accessed in August 1998) because the ADAM data are no longer available for public access online.

32. Black, Hispanic, and white marijuana positive rates were respectively 39.7, 34.1, and 35.2 percent combining males and females across all sites in 1996. My computations based on National Institute of Justice 1998 as in note 3.

33. Computation based on Bureau of Justice Statistics 1999b, table 1.26, indicates that among prisoners newly sentenced to federal prison for drug offenses in 1996, only 7.5 percent were sentenced for possessory offenses. Similarly, among defendants charged with drug felonies and sentenced to prison in state courts in 1996, 68 percent were sentenced for trafficking offenses. (Among state court sentences to jails as opposed to prisons, 56 percent are for trafficking; at the state level, 35 percent of felony drug convictions go to prison, 37 percent to jail and 28 percent to straight probation.) Computations based on Bureau of Justice Statistics 1999c, 3–4. Some convictions for possession are negotiated dispositions of trafficking cases, so that these data probably understate the trafficking share of cases.

34. The Sentencing Project (Mauer and Huling 1995) estimates that in 1995 32.2 percent of black males aged 20–29 were under criminal justice system supervision. Federal estimates for age/race/sex subgroups are not available for all correctional populations, so this estimate is rough.

35. Trend data from the Federal Bureau of Prisons online at www.bop.gov, accessed Dec. 31, 1999.

36. See FBI 1997, tables 70 and 31. Nationwide, cities of over 250,000 have 4.0 law enforcement employees per 1,000 inhabitants as against 3.3 for suburbs. However, they have 510.3 arrests for violent crimes per 100,000 inhabitants as against 198.7 for suburbs. Thus the big-city police departments make over twice as many arrests for violent crimes per employee. This comparison is not perfect because the FBI reporting universe for employee data differs from that for arrest data.
37. Printout provided on Aug. 20, 1998, by FBI, Criminal Justice Information Services Division: analysis of 1996 arrests by race for detailed drug offenses. The data do not differentiate Hispanic and non-Hispanic ethnicity.
38. Vaillant 1995. Vaillant's study focuses on alcoholism; we lack lifecycle studies of the problems associated with illegal drug use.
39. In the 1996 Household Survey, those admitting past-year use of illegal drugs numbered 23.2 million. Only 2.2 million of them admitted being arrested in the past year and only 6.3 million admitted ever having been arrested. Those admitting past-year use of alcohol numbered 138.9 million; among them only 3.2 million admitted arrest in the past year and only 14.9 million admitted ever having been arrested. SAMHSA 1998b accessed online as in note 3.

References

Brownsberger, W. 1997a. "Prevalence of Frequent Cocaine Use in Urban Poverty Areas." *Contemporary Drug Problems* 24(2): 349–371.

———. 1997b. "Profile of Anti-Drug Law Enforcement in Massachusetts." Princeton: Robert Wood Johnson Foundation.

Bureau of Justice Statistics. 1997. *Prisoners in 1996.* Washington.

———. 1998. *Prisoners in 1997.* Washington.

———. 1999a. *Prisoners in 1998.* Washington.

———. 1999b. *Correctional Populations in the United States, 1996.* Washington.

———. 1999c. *Felony Sentences in the United States, 1996.* Washington.

Bureau of the Census. 1993. *Poverty in the United States, 1992.* Series P-60–185. Washington.

Chaiken, J., and Chaiken, M. 1990. "Drugs and Predatory Crime." In Tonry and Wilson 1990.

Drug Enforcement Administration. 1996. "The Threat of Heroin to the United States." Statement of Administrator Thomas A. Constantine before the House Subcommittee on National Security, International Affairs and Criminal Justice, Committee on Government Reform and Oversight,

Sept. 19, 1996. Accessed 12/29/99 at www.usdoj.gov/dea/pubs/cngrtest/ct960919.htm

Edlin, B., Irwin, K., Faruque, S., McCoy, C., Word, C., Serrano, Y., Inciardi, J., Bowser, B., Schilling, R., and Holmberg, S. 1994. "Intersecting Epidemics—Crack Cocaine Use and HIV Infection among Inner-City Young Adults." *New England Journal of Medicine* 331: 1422–27.

Everingham, S., and Rydell, C. 1994. *Modelling the Demand for Cocaine.* Santa Monica: Rand.

Fagan, J. 1990. "Intoxication and Aggression." In Tonry and Wilson 1990.

Federal Bureau of Investigation (FBI). 1997. *Uniform Crime Reports for the United States, 1996* (CD-ROM version). Washington.

———. 1999. *Uniform Crime Reports: Crime in the United States, 1997.* Accessed 12/28/99 at www.fbi.gov/ucr/97cius.htm

Flewelling, R., Rachal, J., and Marsden, M. 1992. *Socioeconomic and Demographic Correlates of Drug and Alcohol Use: Findings from the 1988 and 1990 National Household Survey on Drug Abuse* (DHHS Publication no. ADM 92–1906). Rockville, Md.: National Institute on Drug Abuse.

Harrison, L., Backenheimer, M., and Inciardi, J. 1995. *Cannabis Use in the United States: Implications for Policy.* Newark, Del.: Center for Drug and Alcohol Studies. Online at www.frw.uva.nl/cedro/library/Drugs16/usa.html

House of Representatives, Committee on Government Reform and Oversight. 1995. *Effectiveness of the National Drug Control Strategy and the Status of the Drug War.* Hearings, March 9 and April 6, 1995.

Johnson, R., Gerstein, D., Ghadialy, R., and Choy, W. 1996. *Trends in the Incidence of Drug Use in the United States, 1919–1992.* Rockville, Md.: National Clearing House for Alcohol and Drug Information.

Johnston, L., O'Malley, P., and Bachman, J. 1999. "Drug Trends in 1999 Are Mixed." Ann Arbor: University of Michigan News and Information Services. Accessed 12/26/99 at www.monitoringthefuture.org

Maguire, K., and Pastore, A., eds. 1997. *Sourcebook of Criminal Justice Statistics.* Accessed 7/28/98 at www.albany.edu/sourcebook

Massachusetts Supreme Judicial Court, Substance Abuse Project Task Force. 1995. *A Matter of Just Treatment: Substance Abuse and the Courts.*

Mauer, M., and Huling, T. 1995. *Young Black Americans and the Criminal Justice System: Five Years Later.* Washington: The Sentencing Project.

National Institute on Drug Abuse (NIDA). 1996. *National Survey Results on Drug Use from the Monitoring the Future Study, 1975–1995,* Vol. I: *Secondary School Students.* NIH Publication 96–4139. Washington: Government Printing Office.

———. 1997. *National Survey Results on Drug Use from the Monitoring the Future Study, 1975–1995,* Vol. II: *College Students and Young*

Adults. NIH Publication 98–4140. Washington: Government Printing Office.

――――. 1999. *National Survey Results on Drug Use from the Monitoring the Future Study, 1975–1998,* Vol. I: *Secondary School Students.* NIH Publication 99–4660. Washington: Government Printing Office.

National Institute of Justice. 1998. Drug Use Forecasting in 24 Cities in the United States, 1987–1996 [computer file]. ICPSR version. Ann Arbor: Inter-university Consortium for Political and Social Research [distributor]. This source is no longer available for online calculation.

――――. 1999a. *Arrestee Drug Abuse Monitoring Program: 1998 Annual Report on Adult and Juvenile Arrestees.* Washington.

――――. 1999b. *1998 Annual Report on Cocaine Use among Arrestees.* Washington.

――――. 1999c. *1998 Annual Report on Heroin Use among Arrestees.* Washington.

――――. 1999d. *1998 Annual Report on Marijuana Use among Arrestees.* Washington.

Office of National Drug Control Policy (ONDCP). 1994. *The National Drug Control Strategy 1994.* Washington: The White House.

――――. 1996. *The National Drug Control Strategy 1996.* Washington: The White House.

――――. 1998. *The National Drug Control Strategy 1998.* Washington: The White House.

――――. 1999. *The National Drug Control Strategy 1999.* Washington: The White House.

Ratner, M., ed. 1992. *Crack Pipe as Pimp: An Ethnographic Investigation of Sex-for-Crack Exchanges.* New York: Lexington Books, Macmillan.

Reardon, J. 1993. *The Drug Use Forecasting Study: Measuring Drug Use in a "Hidden" Population.* Washington: National Institute of Justice.

Reuter, P., MacCoun, R., and Murphy, P. 1990. *Money from Crime: A Study of the Economics of Drug Dealing in Washington, D.C.* Santa Monica: Rand.

Rhodes, W. 1993. "Synthetic Estimation Applied to the Prevalence of Drug Use." *Journal of Drug Issues* 23(2): 297–321.

Rhodes, W., Langenbahn, S., Kling, R., and Scheiman, P. 1997. "What America's Users Spend on Illegal Drugs: 1988–1995." White paper prepared for the Office of National Drug Control Policy, available at www.whitehousedrugpolicy.gov

Rydell, C., and Everingham, S. 1994. *Controlling Cocaine: Supply versus Demand Programs.* Santa Monica: Rand.

Saner, H., MacCoun, R., and Reuter, P. 1996. "On the Ubiquity of Drug Selling among Youthful Offenders in Washington, D.C., 1985–1991:

Age Period or Cohort Effect." *Journal of Quantitative Criminology* 11(4): 337–362.

Simeone, R., Rhodes, W., Hunt, D., and Truitt, L. 1997. "A Plan for Estimating the Number of 'Hardcore' Drug Users in the United States: Preliminary Findings." Cambridge, Mass.: Abt Associates.

Substance Abuse and Mental Health Services Administration (SAMHSA). 1996. *Advance Report no. 17: Preliminary Estimates from the Drug Abuse Warning Network, 1995.* Rockville, Md.: National Clearing House for Alcohol and Drug Information.

———. 1998a. *National Household Survey on Drug Abuse, Main Findings: 1996.* Rockville, Md.: National Clearing House for Alcohol and Drug Information.

———. 1998b. National Household Survey on Drug Abuse, 1996 [computer file]. ICPSR version. Ann Arbor: Inter-university Consortium for Political and Social Research [distributor].

———. 1998c. *National Household Survey on Drug Abuse, Population Estimates: 1997.* Rockville, Md.: National Clearing House for Alcohol and Drug Information. Accessed 12/28/99 at www.health.org/pubs/97hhspe/-popes106

———. 1999a. *National Household Survey on Drug Abuse, Population Estimates: 1998.* Rockville, Md.: National Clearing House for Alcohol and Drug Information.

———. 1999b. Summary of Findings from the 1998 National Survey on Drug Abuse. Rockville, Md.: National Clearing House for Alcohol and Drug Information.

———. 1999c. *Prevalence of Substance Use among Racial and Ethnic Subgroups in the United States.* Accessed 12/26/99 at samhsa-ext1.samhsa.gov/oas/NHSDA/Ethnic/Httoc.htm

———. 1999d. *National Household Survey on Drug Abuse, Main Findings: 1997.* Rockville, Md.: National Clearing House for Alcohol and Drug Information. Accessed 12/27/99 at www.samhsa.gov/oas/NHSDA/1997Main

———. 1999e. National Household Survey on Drug Abuse, 1997 [computer file]. ICPSR version. Ann Arbor: Inter-university Consortium for Political and Social Research [distributor].

———. 1999f. *Mid-Year 1998 Preliminary Emergency Department Data from the Drug Abuse Warning Network.* Rockville, Md.: National Clearing House for Alcohol and Drug Information.

———. 1999g. *Treatment Episode Data Set (TEDS): 1992–1997.* Rockville, Md.: National Clearing House for Alcohol and Drug Information. Accessed 12/29/99 at www.samhsa.gov/oas

Tonry, M. 1995. *Malign Neglect: Race, Crime and Punishment in America.* New York: Oxford University Press.

Tonry, M., and Wilson, J., eds. 1990. *Drugs and Crime: Crime and Justice, a Review of Research.* Vol. 13. Chicago: University of Chicago Press.

Vaillant, G. 1995. *Natural History of Alcoholism Revisited.* Cambridge, Mass.: Harvard University Press.

Walinsky, A. 1995. "The Crisis of Public Order." *Atlantic Monthly,* July.

Washton, A. 1987. "Cocaine: Drug Epidemic of the 80s." In D. Allen, ed., *The Cocaine Crisis* (New York: Plenum).

Is Addiction a Chronic, Relapsing Disease?   3

Gene M. Heyman

Addiction is widely considered to be a chronic, relapsing disease. For instance, in an editorial in *Science,* we read that addiction is a "chronic relapsing disease of the nervous system" (Bloom 1997). In a companion article to that editorial, the director of the National Institute on Drug Abuse likens addiction to Alzheimer's disease and schizophrenia, disorders that have no cure (Leshner 1997). And in an article in *Time* magazine, addiction is coupled with diabetes and hypertension, two diseases that likewise are chronic (Nash 1997).

However, research shows that many addicts recover. Among a group of inner-city heroin addicts in St. Louis, all claimed to have kicked their addiction by the time they were in their thirties (Robins and Murphy 1967). Although the sample in the St. Louis study was small, the result may be representative of most of those who become addicted. Large-scale epidemiological surveys reveal that there are millions of recovered smokers, alcoholics, and drug addicts (e.g. Robins and Regier 1991; Schelling 1992). In-depth studies of small populations of cocaine addicts (Waldorf, Reinarman, and Murphy 1991) and heroin addicts (Biernacki 1986) tell much the same story: several years of heavy drug use followed by an apparently enduring period of abstinence or controlled drug use. Possibly these studies are misleading, reflecting biased methods rather than the nature of addiction. On the other hand, perhaps the claim that addiction is a chronic, relapsing disease is misleading. The issue is an empirical one, and we now know enough about addiction to settle it.

The question of whether addiction is a chronic disorder is central to policy, treatment, and research. For instance, some male heroin addicts commit crimes at rates that approach one a day during periods of heavy drug use (e.g. Ball, Shaffer, and Nurco 1983). If addiction is typically chronic, then these men can be expected to commit scores if not hundreds of crimes every time they are released from prison. However, if addiction wanes with age or with the responsibilities that usually accompany age, it would be wrong to set sentences on the expectation of a lifelong pattern of drug-related crime. Clinicians who treat addicts face a different set of problems. Are they misleading their clients when they endorse the idea that recovery is the norm or when they endorse the idea that relapse is the norm? Presumably the ability to remain abstinent can be influenced by information about relapse rates, and it would be irresponsible to tell an addict that he or she had a chronic disease if in fact this was not true.

Neuroscientists who study drug-induced changes in the brain often identify these changes as the substrates of a chronic, relapsing disease, without mention of the reports indicating that recovery is the rule. That is, even in the scientific community there is not a general awareness of the conflicting findings regarding addiction relapse rates. This is unfortunate. Researchers may be assuming irreversible damage when in fact the brain changes are temporary and/or readily reversible by means of environmentally induced experiences. More generally, the brain may be a good deal more dynamic and plastic than assumed in current biological accounts of addiction. In short, whether we are judges, clinicians, or scientists, we need to know if addicts typically recover, or if "once an addict, always an addict."

Much of the research reviewed in this chapter was made possible by advances in the ability to reliably diagnose psychiatric cases. In the late 1970s the American Psychiatric Association revised its criteria for identifying psychiatric disorders. The goal was to ensure higher inter-rater reliability. By this standard, the new nosology (APA 1980) was a success (e.g. Spitzer and Forman 1979; Spitzer, Forman, and Nee 1979). On average, reliability increased by about 50 percent, and for substance-use disorders reliability scores were usually above 80 percent. An immediate consequence of diagnostic progress was scientific progress, especially in the area of psychiatric epidemiology. For instance, recent estimates of national frequencies of psychiatric disorders often agree within a few percentage points, whereas earlier epidemiological research produced notoriously inconsistent results (e.g. Sandifer et al. 1968). Consequently, a good starting point for the investigation of relapse rates is the American Psychiatric Association's (APA) criteria for identifying addiction.

The most recent version of the APA diagnostic manual (1994) defines addiction ("substance dependence") as a "cluster of cognitive, behavioral, and physiological symptoms indicating that the individual continues to use the substance despite significant substance-related problems." Features of the disorder include tolerance, withdrawal, and loss of control over drug use. Loss of control, which is also referred to as "compulsive drug use," means such things as taking more of a drug than was initially intended, persistently trying and failing to curtail or quit taking drugs, and spending less time in conventional activities in order to pursue drug use. Tolerance and withdrawal are neither necessary nor sufficient for the diagnosis, and although the same can be said for loss of control, it is this feature of addiction that has been most emphasized by clinicians and scientists. "Compulsive" use leads to the adverse consequences that typify addiction and also to tolerance and withdrawal, and "compulsive" use is what is so hard to explain. For example, purchasing illicit drugs in the amounts required to maintain addiction requires planning and guile. And yet this pursuit, according to many clinicians, is "compulsive" and "out of control." But how can behavior that is planned also be "out of control"? (At the end of this chapter, this contradiction will be resolved. I will argue that "compulsive drug use" is better described as "ambivalent" drug use. The difference is important. Ambivalent users can be persuaded to stop, compulsive users cannot.)

Relapse Rates

The View from the Clinic

One of the major sources of information on addiction is research on treatment. The typical finding is that within a year or so of leaving the clinic the patient has resumed drug use (e.g. Stephens and Cottrell 1972; Vaillant 1966; Wasserman et al. 1998). Figure 3.1 shows some often-cited results. On the x-axis is time since the completion of treatment. On the y-axis is the percentage of patients who resumed drug use. Despite treatment, within 12 months most addicts had resumed

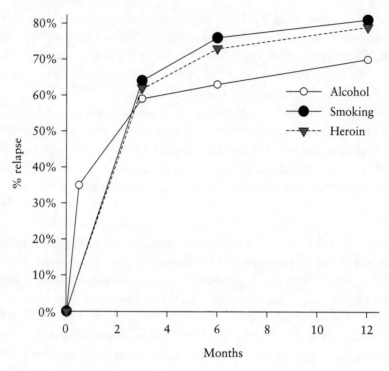

Figure 3.1. Relapse rates over time after treatment: alcohol, tobacco, and heroin. Source: Hunt, Barnett, and Branch 1971.

drug use. Other studies show the same pattern (e.g. Brecher 1972). For example, in a text for clinicians (Thombs 1994), the author emphasizes an outcome study that found 90 percent relapse rates for all substance-disorder patients, and he ends the section on relapse with a warning to the intended readers (future clinicians) to remain skeptical of any program that claims to have devised a successful program for treating addiction. The simplest interpretation of Figure 3.1 is that addiction is indeed a chronic, relapsing disorder. However, there is a well-known methodological problem in clinic-based outcome research. Individuals who suffer from more than one disorder are more likely to seek treatment ("Berkson's bias"). For instance, addicts who also suffer from depression or AIDS are the ones most likely to be the subjects in clinic research. This may or may not make a difference. If pharmacology alone predicted relapse rates, then comorbidity would not matter. However, if general health also mattered, then clinic populations could greatly overestimate relapse rates, especially if most addicts did not seek treatment.

Recovery and Relapse in Non-clinic Heroin Addicts

One way to avoid Berkson's bias is to select subjects independently of whether they end up in treatment. The next two studies take this approach. In both, the subjects were heroin addicts.

Robins and Murphy (1967) studied the behavioral and familial antecedents of heroin addiction in African-American men who had grown up in St. Louis right after World War II. The men were identified on the basis of their elementary school registration forms, not drug use. While they were in their late teens and early twenties, some 13 percent of the sample experimented with heroin, and of this subgroup, about 75 percent became addicted. However, as they approached their late twenties and early thirties, they stopped using heroin. For the year prior to the interview, 84 percent claimed no heroin use, and the other 16 percent said they used occasionally but were not addicted. That is, according to self-report, the recovery rate was 100 percent. Official records support these results. Two-thirds of the men were known to the Federal Bureau of Narcotics, and of these, 74 percent did not have a record of heroin use in the five years prior to the study. Robins and Murphy add that according to health and judicial records, the men typically told the truth about their drug-use history (and there was no obvious advantage in misleading the researchers).

The second non-clinic study involves American servicemen who began using opiates (usually heroin) while in Vietnam. More than 40 percent used heroin at least once. Of those who tried the drug at least five times, about 90 percent went on to become regular users. In 1971 several thousand soldiers were returning from Vietnam each month. Given the clinic relapse rates (see Figure 3.1), it was widely, and sensibly, believed that a domestic heroin epidemic was imminent. President Nixon requested a study of the problem, and Lee Robins, who had directed the St. Louis study, was asked to head the project. She and her colleagues collected data on drug use in a sample of 898 men who were scheduled to be discharged in September 1971 after serving in Vietnam (Robins, Helzer, and Davis 1975).

Of those who became regular heroin users, about 70 percent met the study's criteria for addiction (withdrawal symptoms and difficulty quitting). But one year after returning to the United States, 95 percent were no longer regular users (ibid.), and three years later the remission rate was still close to 90 percent (Robins et al. 1980). This dramatic decrease in heroin use was not simply a matter of heroin's becoming less available. About 50 percent of those addicted in Vietnam had tried heroin after returning home, yet they did not resume regular use of the drug.

Unfortunately, the authors provide little information about the recovery process. We can surmise that it was aided by a wide array of informal methods, as only 6 percent of the Vietnam opiate users went to drug treatment centers. (They were eligible for care at VA hospitals.) Figure 3.2 shows the Vietnam results and those of a typical clinic study. They are virtually mirror images of one another. Addicts in conventional treatment facilities typically returned to drug use; addicts who did not seek treatment typically recovered.

The clinic-based and non-clinic-based studies could not have produced more discrepant results. Nevertheless, the differences may be illusory. For example, the St. Louis men and the Vietnam enlistees may have been opiate users but not real opiate addicts. This distinction has a precedent. Some heroin users are able to regulate their intake so that their drug use does not interfere with other aspects of their life ("chippers"). For instance, a common pattern for the controlled heroin user is to restrict use to Saturdays, thereby ensuring that periods of intoxication do not interfere with work and allowing a day for recovery (Zinberg et al. 1977). Thus we should evaluate the possibility that the subjects in the two non-clinic studies were heroin users but not really heroin addicts.

The St. Louis men typically injected heroin for several years or more, 50 percent were sentenced to federal hospitals for addiction, and almost all were known to public officials as addicts. They were recognized by their peers and the authorities as street addicts. If the Vietnam sample is restricted to those who injected heroin more than once a week, the recovery rates are still more than 80 percent. The

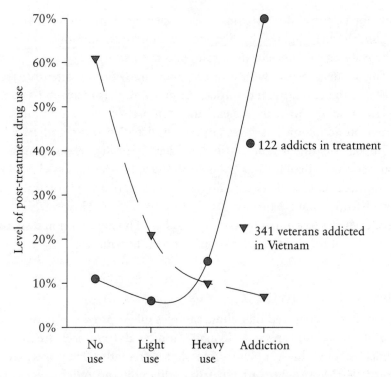

Figure 3.2. Levels of heroin use for addicts in treatment and veterans return-ing from Vietnam. Sources: Stephens and Cottrell 1972; Robins 1993.

same holds for men who kept using heroin even though they knew that an opiate-positive urine test might delay their departure for home (Robins, Helzer, and Davis 1975). Thus the high recovery rates in these two non-clinic populations do not appear to be due to a too lib-eral definition of addiction.

A more important methodological issue is whether the recovery rate results are representative of addicts in general. Although 10 per-cent of the St. Louis sample became heroin addicts, this amounts to only 22 men. In the Vietnam research there were more subjects (386 opiate users), but their experience may not be relevant to conditions elsewhere. In Vietnam, heroin was cheap, use typically went unpun-ished, and the men were caught in a bitter, highly controversial war. Some might argue that this situation is too unusual to provide lessons about the nature of addiction. (On the other hand, these conditions may not be too different from those experienced by addicts living in neighborhoods blighted by abandoned buildings, shooting galleries, and grudging tolerance of drug sales and use.)

This chapter began with a discrepancy: addiction is often referred to as a chronic, relapsing disorder, yet many addicts recover. The data reviewed so far provide a neat and comprehensive resolution. Research on addiction has been largely restricted to those addicts who end up in treatment; addicts in treatment typically relapse within a year or so (e.g. Brecher 1972; Thombs 1994; Wasserman et al. 1998). In contrast, those addicts who do not end up in treatment typically recover (Robins and Murphy 1967; Robins 1993). However, so far there are only two non-clinic-based studies. The next section tests the generality of the treatment-vs.-nontreatment hypothesis.

Large National Surveys in Community Samples

Researchers recognized that clinic samples might provide a biased picture of addiction, especially if many addicts did not seek treatment. Clinicians saw this problem somewhat differently. They were concerned that those who suffered from addiction and other psychiatric disorders were not getting the treatment they needed. Both issues pointed to the need for a survey of mental health problems in a large, representative sample. In the late 1970s circumstances fell into place to make this sort of survey possible.

Shortly following her husband's inauguration, Rosalynn Carter, wife of President Jimmy Carter, convened a meeting of mental health experts at the White House. The experts recommended a nationwide survey of psychiatric disorders, including addiction (Regier et al. 1984). The National Institutes of Health sponsored the research, now known as the Epidemiological Catchment Area Study (ECA), and the results were summarized in a book published in 1991 (Robins and Regier 1991).

The ECA selected subjects from five major metropolitan areas, independently of their treatment history. Because of the size of the effort (nearly 20,000 subjects), the interviewers (about 200) were not professional clinicians but a specially trained lay staff. Their primary instrument was a questionnaire designed so that the answers could be classified in terms of the recently revised and field-tested American Psychiatric Association diagnostic categories (APA 1980).

For most diagnoses, the reliability between lay interviewers and psychiatrists was as good as that between different psychiatrists (Helzer et al. 1985), and the average number of symptoms per case was virtually identical for lay and professionally trained interviewers (Helzer, Spitzagel, and McEvoy 1987). In addition, some ten years after the ECA survey there was a second large, nationwide evaluation of psychiatric health in community samples. This survey, known as the National Comorbidity Study (NCS), provides a convenient check on the reliability of the ECA results. Other methodological issues, such as whether the sample population was representative of addicts in general or whether the interviewees accurately reported their drug use, will be addressed later.

Figure 3.3 shows the ECA and NCS estimates of remission rates for addiction and other psychiatric disorders. In the ECA study, remission was defined as no symptoms for the year just prior to the interview. In the NCS study, which included about 8,000 respondents, the criterion for remission was anything less than the minimum set of symptoms for establishing a diagnosis. That is, the ECA criteria for remission were more conservative. In both studies substance-use disorders had the highest remission rates. According to the NCS results, 76 percent of all of those with a lifetime diagnosis were not addicted for a year or more prior to the interview. According to the ECA respondents, the remission rate was 59 percent. For other psychiatric diagnoses the remission rates were lower, and in much closer agreement. Indeed, if substance-use disorder is not included, then the average difference in relapse rates for the NCS and ECA surveys is only 2 percent. One interpretation of this pattern of findings is that the ECA and NCS used similar criteria for identifying active and recovered cases for every disorder but addiction. In support of this interpretation, when the NCS researchers use the ECA criteria for addiction, the difference in remission rates shrinks to less than 5 percent (Warner et al. 1995). Thus the "discrepancy" appears to reflect the faithful application of the diagnostic criteria, rather than unreliable instruments.

Although both surveys found that substance-use disorders had the highest remission rates, this result requires further analysis. The NCS

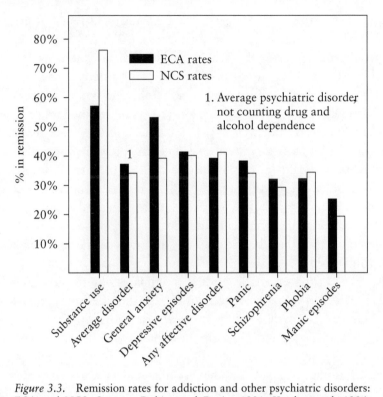

Figure 3.3. Remission rates for addiction and other psychiatric disorders: ECA and NCS. Sources: Robins and Regier 1991; Kessler et al. 1994; Warner et al. 1995.

and ECA typically did not differentiate between the various illicit drugs. Results for opiate, stimulant, and marijuana use were averaged together, as if these drugs were sufficiently similar to be considered a single category. However, they have markedly different pharmacological and behavioral effects, which may well lead to quite different relapse rates. In particular, many experts believe that the consequences of frequent marijuana use are significantly less debilitating than the consequences of frequent stimulant and opiate use. Thus the survey results on relapse may be accurate for marijuana but not for opiates and stimulants. Figure 3.4 addresses this issue. (It is based on the one table in the ECA summary that organizes drug-use statistics by drug class).

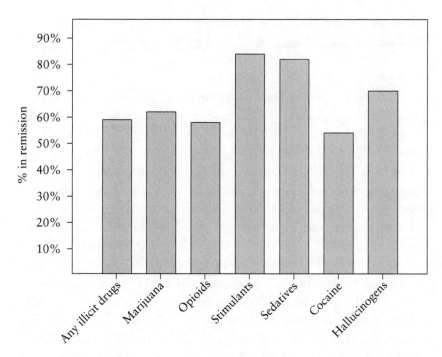

Figure 3.4. Remission rates by type of illicit drug. Source: ECA data, Anthony and Helzer 1991, table 6.4.

As expected, cocaine and opiates had the lowest recovery rates, but the more important point is that for the major illicit addictive drugs, the remission rates were quite similar and reasonably well represented by the average value. Marijuana users did not skew the results.

The national survey results lead to the same conclusion as the St. Louis and Vietnam findings. Most addicts recover, but this is only apparent if the addicts are selected independently of their treatment history. An immediate implication is that addiction is reversible. Before addressing this issue, I will review data on the duration of addiction. Low relapse rates suggest a relatively short duration. However, this is a logical point, and the data could turn out differently. The duration results will also provide a kind of check on the relapse findings. If addiction has the lowest relapse rate of any psychiatric disorder, then it should, all else being equal, have the shortest duration of any psychiatric disorder. But the claims published in *Science* and *Time* that introduced this chapter suggest a quite different outcome.

Duration

The ECA report provides estimates of the duration of addiction for active and remitted cases. From these two pieces of information plus the remission rates just reviewed, it is possible to get some idea of how long addiction typically lasts.

The ECA researchers identified the onset of a disorder as the initial expression of one or more symptoms (rather than when the full case criteria were first met). For individuals who met the criteria for abuse and/or dependence at the time of the interview (current addicts), the average time since onset was 6.1 years and the median time was between 4 and 5 years (Anthony and Helzer 1991). For individuals in remission for 3 or more years (no symptoms related to drug use for at least 3 years), the average time from onset to remission was 2.7 years and the median duration was between 1 and 2 years. When the mean and median of a distribution markedly differ, the distribution is not bell-shaped but asymmetrical. When this is true, the median is the more representative population measure. Thus for recovered addicts (no symptoms for three years), addiction typically lasted less than two years.

These estimates are based on interviews, and there were no independent checks as to their validity. They could be accurate, but they also could reflect the manner in which questions were worded, the tendency, when providing a history, to reconstruct the past in terms of current circumstances, and normal difficulties in accurately remembering subtle changes in behavior, especially ones that took place gradually over an extended period.

One way to correct for the errors inherent in retrospective research is to use relative rather than absolute measures. For instance, under the assumption that errors and distortions are more or less equally likely across the different disorders, the ratio of the remembered duration of one disorder to the remembered duration of another disorder should reflect the actual ratios. Figure 3.5 is motivated by this logic. It shows the ECA estimates of duration for the more frequent psychiatric disorders.

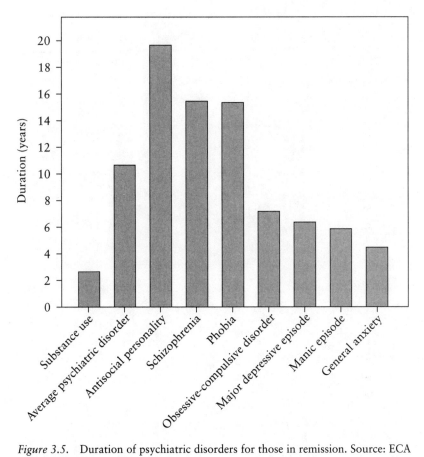

Figure 3.5. Duration of psychiatric disorders for those in remission. Source: ECA estimates, Robins and Regier 1991.

Substance-use disorder had the shortest duration, and the differences are substantial: in remitted cases, the average psychiatric disorder lasted about four times longer than did addiction, and schizophrenia lasted about seven times longer.

Despite the methodological problems in estimating duration, there are reasons to have some confidence in the results shown in this figure. First, there is an inverse relationship between duration and remission, which is the simplest possible relationship. Second, the estimated durations agree with clinical experience. Those that were longer, such as schizophrenia, clinicians find least tractable, and those that were shorter, such as anxiety disorders, are thought to be more treatable.

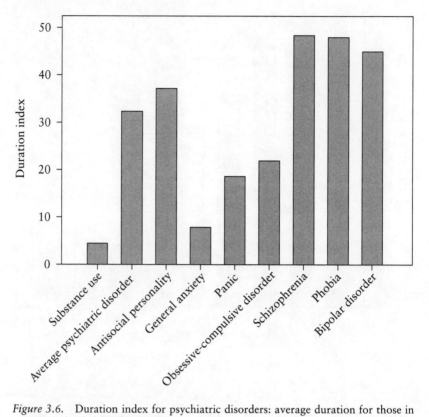

Figure 3.6. Duration index for psychiatric disorders: average duration for those in remission divided by the percentage of cases in remission. Source: calculated from data in Robins and Regier 1991.

However, Figure 3.5 has a serious limitation. It includes only cases that were in remission at the time of the ECA interview. Active cases were excluded (and they are likely to last longer). A simple way to correct for this omission is to factor in remission rates. For instance, disorders with higher proportions of active cases must last longer, all else being equal. Figure 3.6 reflects this line of reasoning. It shows the average duration for those in remission divided by the percentage of cases in remission. For instance, if half the cases were in remission, "duration" was doubled.

When both remitted and active cases are included in the same measure, the relative duration of addiction shrinks even further. For example, now the "duration" of addiction is less than one-sixth that of the average psychiatric disorder and less than one-tenth that of schizophrenia. (Individual biographies and survey data show that addiction often comes to an end, so it is sensible to ask how long it lasts. In contrast, for many other psychiatric disorders the notion of an endpoint is really not sensible, at least for a large portion of the victims. Schizophrenia and depression are often lifelong, chronic maladies. This observation does not make the figures meaningless; rather it reinforces the point they make: among psychiatric disorders, addiction is usually the outlier.)

Summary of Relapse, Remission, and Duration Results

According to the idea that addiction is a chronic disorder, when addicts go on the wagon, they are soon to fall off. In support of this view are the results from clinic outcome studies showing high relapse rates (e.g. Wasserman et al. 1998). However, studies that did not use clinic populations (e.g. Robins and Murphy 1967; Robins, Helzer, and Davis 1975) showed just the opposite result: addicts recovered. Large-scale epidemiological surveys in which subjects were selected independent of treatment history showed the same pattern as the nonclinic research. Of all the psychiatric disorders, addiction had the highest remission rate and the shortest duration. Thus, once you sample addicts in a nonbiased manner, addiction no longer appears to be a chronic, relapsing disorder.

However, the survey findings do not imply that the clinic results are invalid or unimportant. Rather, they show that there are large individual differences. Although most addicts recover, many struggle for years, cycling back and forth between sobriety and heavy drug use (Brecher 1972; Vaillant 1992). To understand addiction, it is necessary to understand why the route to recovery is so varied. The most obvious starting point is "Why are addicts who seek treatment more likely to relapse than those who do not seek treatment?"

Addicts Who Seek Treatment vs. Those Who Do Not

The contrast between clinic relapse rates and the ECA and NCS estimates of relapse implies that most addicts do not seek treatment and suggests that the correlates of the differences between those who do and do not seek treatment will provide clues to the factors that deter recovery. The ECA data support the logic. Approximately 70 percent of those with a lifetime diagnosis of substance-use disorder were not treated for drug use. However, differences between treated and untreated addicts have been little studied. Other than two reports from researchers at Yale University, there is little published research on this important topic.

The available results will be organized in terms of three factors: pharmacological history; consequences of drug use, such as arrests; and individual traits, such as psychiatric history. (It is likely that those who do not end up in treatment centers get help from friends, family, and co-workers. This, though, does not rule out the possibility that "treated" and "untreated" addicts truly differ.)

Pharmacological history.   It is reasonable to suppose that those who do not seek treatment are relatively new users, who have not been as exposed to drugs as those in treatment. Some research supports this view (e.g. Chitwood and Chitwood 1981; Graeven and Graeven 1983). However, authors of more recent studies (e.g. Carroll and Rounsaville 1992) point out that earlier researchers did not use field-tested diagnostic criteria or attempt to ensure that both populations met some minimum threshold for addiction. The criticism appears to be valid: a different picture emerges in the two Yale studies, in which both treated and untreated populations were selected according to the APA diagnostic criteria (Rounsaville and Kleber 1985; Carroll and Rounsaville 1992). One was with heroin addicts, the other with cocaine addicts. The treated subjects were from the clinic, the untreated subjects were contacted by word of mouth. In these studies both treated and untreated individuals "qualified" as addicts according to the APA criteria.

Level of drug use.   Cocaine addicts who did not utilize clinics exceeded the clinic cocaine addicts on all measures of drug use. In particular, they were more likely to use a wide array of addictive drugs. The same pattern held for heroin addicts. Both treated and untreated addicts had been using heroin daily for about six years, but the non-treatment group reported more alcohol and marijuana use. Thus the two most complete studies fail to provide evidence that pharmacological history distinguishes treated and untreated addicts.

Adverse consequences of drug use.   Treatment-seeking cocaine addicts reported significantly higher levels of recent depression and anxiety, and significantly greater negative consequences of cocaine use in relation to family, friends, and work (Carroll and Rounsaville 1992). Among heroin addicts, those who sought clinic help had more severe drug-related problems in respect to social interactions and significantly more arrests for drug possession and sales. (The "untreated" addicts obtained about 70 percent of the income for heroin by illegal acts and reported that they had been engaged in criminal activity for profit in about 14 out of the last 30 days.) In summarizing the findings for opiate addicts, Rounsaville and Kleber (1985) write, "Overall, the findings seem to indicate that while heavy drug use per se may not be a primary motivation to seek treatment, social, legal, and psychological problems that are acutely associated with the drug use may provide the incentive to apply for help." Rounsaville and Kleber's point is that the two groups did not differ in regard to their level of drug use, but did differ in regard to the number of problems they reported, and that many of these problems were immediate consequences of drug use.

Individual differences.   The Yale studies show that similar pharmacological histories did not lead to similar outcomes. This implies that individual differences mediate many critical drug effects. Individual differences in drug metabolism are likely to play an important role, and Rounsaville and Kleber (1985) stress individual differences in social support. However, the best evidence for differences between treated and untreated addicts comes from the study of co-occurring psychiatric disorders ("comorbidity").

Regier et al. (1990) write that the expected likelihood of a non-drug-related psychiatric disorder among addicts in the ECA sample, assuming no increased risk, was 22 percent. In contrast, the observed frequency was more than twice as great, 53 percent. The increased liability varied by drug class. About 50 percent of marijuana abusers met the criteria for an additional psychiatric diagnosis, whereas the proportions were 65 percent and 76 percent for opiate and cocaine disorders, respectively. However, the largest difference was between those who sought treatment and those who did not. For those who did not seek treatment, the prevalence of other psychiatric disorders was about 29 percent, not too different from the expected value. Among treatment seekers, the prevalence of other mental disorders was more than twice as great, 64 percent (and almost three times greater than the expected value). Thus the persistence of addiction was closely tied to the presence of a co-occurring disorder.

The ECA results are supported by smaller, clinic-based studies. In a comparison of drug users who signed up for treatment versus those who signed up to be experimental subjects (Montoya et al. 1995), the treatment seekers scored higher on eight of nine measures of psychopathology (and the non-treatment group was in the "normal" range on all measures). In the work done at Yale, treatment seekers were significantly more likely to be suffering from depression.

Why do co-occurring psychiatric disorders deter recovery from addiction? The correlational structure across disorders is complex. Addicts show elevated risks for almost all diagnoses, with the correlations for conduct disorder, bipolar disorder, and depression ranking highest (Regier et al. 1990). This pattern supports the idea that people who use addictive drugs to medicate themselves are more likely to become addicted (e.g. Khantzian 1985). Also, psychiatric disorders may undermine activities that would normally provide a compelling alternative to the addictive drug. For example, addicts who become involved in athletics, hobbies, and clubs are more likely to successfully abstain from drug use (Waldorf 1983). Unfortunately, those with psychiatric disorders are less likely to join groups and take up hobbies. Thus, with too much time on their hands, the psychiatric patients turn to addictive drugs. This point is similar to the self-medication hypothesis, but differs in that drug use fills a void rather than functions as medication for a specific disorder.

That most addicts recover has not been widely appreciated, and thus little has been written about differences between those who successfully abstain and those who do not. However, the available evidence is consistent. Pharmacological history did not make any obvious difference in recovery rates, whereas individual differences in psychiatric history did. This is not to say that drug pharmacology is unimportant. For example, it is possible that the biological effects of addictive drugs are quite different as a function of additional psychiatric disorders, and, as noted in the conclusion of this chapter, pharmacological treatments for addiction are of proven worth and should be further developed. Nevertheless, the simplest account of the available data is that recovery from addiction is significantly influenced by nonpharmacological factors.

Is Addiction a Disease?

There are several senses in which it is legitimate to call addiction a disease. According to one dictionary, a disease is a "departure from a normal condition in a negative way that can be identified by a characteristic group of signs or symptoms." The definition applies. Most consider addiction a departure from the norm, and it can be reliably identified by clinicians. However, by the same criteria, behaviors that we are more likely to call bad habits become diseases. For instance, there are people who spend an abnormally large amount of time watching television—about eight to twelve hours a day (Goleman 1990). At the end of their television marathon, they feel bad about how much time they have wasted and state that they wish they had spent the time more productively. Nevertheless, the next day they are in front of the television again. Their behavior is excessive and, from their own perspective, deleterious. Thus, by the dictionary definition, excessive television watching is a disease. Similar analyses easily apply to long hours at the office, surfing the net, and the scores of other familiar yet excessive behaviors. But most of us believe these activities are clearly different from having cancer, heart disease, or even diabetes (which has a large behavioral component). In support of this intuition, everyday use of the term "disease" reveals a more discriminating understanding than the dictionary definition. In everyday speech "disease" has two rather specific meanings.

First, many call addiction a disease because some instances can be tied to a biological predisposition and because addictive drugs change the brain (e.g. Lewis 1991; Leshner 1997; Maltzman 1994). However, all goal-oriented behavior is mediated by the brain, and all learned behavior depends on changes in the brain. For example, heritability studies indicate a genetic predisposition for various forms of criminal behavior (Wilson and Herrnstein 1985), and it seems likely that future research will show that certain environmental events alter the brain in ways that increase the likelihood of violence (e.g. Miczek 1999). Thus, by the criterion of "biological basis," all crimes would eventually become diseases. But this would lead to foolish and morally unacceptable policies. For instance, medical hospitalization for crimes such as murder and car theft would violate widely shared ideas of justice and, if consequences count, would prove counterproductive. Thus the idea that a disorder is a disease because it has a biological basis or because it entails brain changes is too crude a standard.

The second colloquial meaning of "disease" is that it is an involuntary, as opposed to a voluntary, disorder. This turns out to be a practical and scientifically defensible distinction. The mechanisms mediating voluntary and involuntary disorders differ, especially in regard to the influence of the central nervous system. Treatments for voluntary and involuntary disorders often differ (it would be cruel to punish tics or hallucinations, but it might be quite helpful and humane to provide corrective incentives for excessive television watchers). And social institutions for the remediation of voluntary and involuntary behavioral problems differ (e.g. "wise men" and "medicine men"). In short, the question of whether addiction is a voluntary or involuntary disorder matters (whereas there should be no question that addiction has a biological basis).

The idea that addicts take drugs involuntarily has been articulately argued by clinicians and researchers. Miller and Chappel (1991), psychiatrists, explained that addicts have a disease because they have lost control over drug use. Jellinek (1960), one of the first to systematically study alcoholism, defined alcoholism as a disease on the basis of loss of control over drinking. More recently, Leshner (1997), the head of the National Institute on Drug Abuse, claimed that repeated ingestion of addictive drugs "turns off" voluntary control of drug use.

However, the idea that a behavior is "out of control" does not seem to automatically qualify it as a disease. The excessive television watchers claimed that their behavior was out of control, and yet most observers would want to distinguish their problems from those of cancer patients, diabetics, schizophrenics, and even addicts. Also, the statement that addicts are unable to control their drug use is not accurate. For example, pack-a-day cigarette smokers meet the DSM criteria for addiction, yet since the Surgeon General's report in 1964 on the health effects of smoking, some 50 million heavy smokers have quit using cigarettes (Schelling 1992). Moreover, most quit on their own, without medical help. If addiction is out-of-control drug use, how is this possible? On the other hand, it is no simple matter to quit an addictive drug. Thus the question of whether addiction is in fact involuntary drug use has remained controversial (e.g. Vuchinich 1996). Part of the problem is that there are no widely agreed upon criteria for identifying voluntary acts.

Criteria for Identifying Voluntary Acts

The distinction between voluntary and involuntary acts pervades the discussion and analysis of behavior. In philosophy and political theory, the distinction is usually made along the lines of conscious intentions (Searle 1983) and/or freedom from authoritarian regimes. In scientific studies of behavior, the criteria have to do with the factors that influence behavior. Some behaviors are elicited by stimulus conditions and are relatively immune to reward and punishment (e.g. reflexes). Other behaviors have no specific eliciting conditions, but instead are learned; their frequency is a function of deprivation and relative reward and punishment. For example, consider the contrast between two simple, topographically similar behaviors, "eye blinks" and "winks."

An eye blink is a "wired-in" behavior that is readily elicited by a directed force to the eye, such as a puff of air. The wiring admits specific eliciting stimuli, but provides few if any inputs for the influence of incentives or payoffs (contingencies). For instance, if a one-dollar incentive failed to inhibit the defensive blink, increases on the order of a hundred or even a thousand would not change this outcome. Consequently, defensive blinks are identified as reflexive as opposed to learned acts.

Winking is topographically similar to blinking, but its determinants (and hence its biology) are quite different. Winks that are reinforced by camaraderie or a shared secret tend to persist; those which are met by derision or disgust tend to fade. That is, rather weak rewards readily influence winking.

In everyday speech, we would say that the person intended to wink, could have done otherwise, or chose to wink. But in all these cases it is possible to make a simpler (and measurable) statement: "winking" is more susceptible to control by consequences than is "blinking." The distinction is not between freedom of the will and determinism or between psychology and biology. Winks and blinks are equally determined and equally biological. However, the biology of the two behaviors differs. The anatomy of winking permits the influence of consequences, whereas the neural basis of blinks supports eliciting stimuli and admits little if any of the effects of contingent consequences.

Voluntary as a Matter of Degree

"Control by consequences" is not, of course, an all-or-none matter. Behaviors vary in the degree to which they are influenced by consequences, and behavioral syndromes differ in their mix of reflexive and learned components. For instance, the tics in Tourette's syndrome or the hallucinations in schizophrenia do not seem to be readily influenced by contingencies, whereas the motor components of obsessive compulsive disorder do show some susceptibility to reward and punishment. Juvenile delinquency clearly has a biological component (given the age and gender correlations), but teenage acting out is probably more susceptible to consequences than are the motor components of obsessive compulsive disorder. In other words, one could construct a continuum in which disorders were ranked in regard to their susceptibility to the influence of various forms of persuasion (benefits, penalties, new information, and the like).

According to this analysis, the questions of whether addiction is a voluntary behavioral disorder or a disease can be rephrased as "To what extent will contingent rewards and punishments (broadly conceived) control drug consumption in addicts?" Again, the issue is not whether addiction has a biological basis or whether drugs change the brain. Rather, the issue is whether the biology of addiction results in a state such that drug consumption is no longer significantly influenced by its consequences. To answer this question, we need to test whether rewards, punishments, new information, and other forms of persuasion significantly influence drug consumption in addicts.

"Compulsive" Drug Use as Ambivalent Drug Use

Recall that the APA diagnostic manual defines addiction as the continued use of drugs despite their adverse consequences. According to the above discussion, this implies that addiction is involuntary. However, the authors of the manual left out a critical fact. A common feature of alcohol, nicotine, stimulants, and opiates is that they provide immediate positive consequences but delayed aversive consequences (withdrawal, penalties for intoxication, health risks, and so on). From this perspective, it is easy to see that addiction may well be a matter of contingencies: large and positive immediate consequences competing with large but delayed aversive consequences for the control of drug consumption. In these terms, addiction is ambivalence, with the decision to use drugs dependent on the temporal horizon. When the temporal frame of reference is relatively short, drug use is preferred; when the temporal frame of reference is relatively long, abstinence is preferred. Thus, what appears to be "compulsive" behavior may actually be a shift in preference, which, in turn, is a function of the temporal horizon at the moment of choice.

The difference between ambivalence and compulsion is important. By definition, a person who is ambivalent can be influenced by incentives, new information, changes in perspective, and all the sorts of acts that come under the general rubric "persuasion." In contrast, compulsive behaviors are, by definition, not influenced by persuasion. For instance, if monetary incentives strongly influenced the frequency of hand washing in a patient with the diagnosis "obsessive compulsive disorder," we would probably decide that the diagnosis was wrong. Note that this example suggests the practical and relative nature of these judgments. Assume for a moment that financial rewards can, in principle, have some effect on "compulsive" hand washing. The degree to which we are willing to call the act compulsive would be likely to depend on the amount of financial reward that was required for ameliorative change. If the amount was too large to have any practical application, then the available contingencies would be useless, and the hand washing would meet the criteria for compulsive behavior. Thus, to determine whether addiction entails ambivalence toward drug use or compulsive drug use, it is necessary to see if addicts can be persuaded to stop using drugs.

Laboratory Tests

There is a small but important series of experiments on whether contingencies can influence drug consumption in addicts. The subjects were long-term alcoholics who sought inpatient treatment for their drinking problems. The basic finding was that contingencies significantly modified drinking. For instance, in one of the more realistic studies, alcoholics were given free "priming" drinks and then offered incentives for not drinking further. Larger priming drinks were more likely to lead to a binge. However, for every priming dose there was an incentive that would promote self-control (see Cohen et al. 1971; Bigelow and Liebson 1972). It is not known whether this experience led to a lasting cure. But the question before us is whether it is possible to persuade an addict to stop using drugs. These data show that under experimental conditions, it is. (Also, according to the reports, the subjects were extremely alcoholic and would have met Jellinek's criteria for loss of control over drinking.)

Natural Experiments: Vietnam

In the United States heroin has socially mediated aversive consequences. In Vietnam many of these aversive consequences were weakened or absent. Prohibitions against heroin were rarely enforced, and users apparently did not think of themselves as "junkies" or criminals. Thus, if addiction is a matter of choice, "simply" returning to the United States should have significantly reduced heroin addiction in the Vietnam enlistees. This is exactly what happened, and the recovery rates were above 80 percent. Of course, the contingencies surrounding drug use were not the only differences between conditions in Vietnam and the United States. The men were at war in a hostile environment. However, the reports suggest that changes in the consequences of drug use played an important role. For example, the men cite heroin's "sordid" reputation and the dangers involved in purchasing the drugs as reasons for quitting.

Historical Changes and Cohort Effects

The social consequences of illicit drug use varied markedly over the course of the twentieth century. Opiates and cocaine were legal in the United States until 1914; during the 1960s and 1970s there was wider acceptance of mind-altering drugs (including cocaine and heroin); and more recently there has been a concerted effort to dissociate addictive drugs from their earlier, positive connotations. Thus, if addiction is influenced by its consequences, there should be marked historical trends, even over rather short periods of time.

Figure 3.7, based on the NCS study, shows drug use and dependence given use (a measure of susceptibility to addiction) in men. The data are organized in terms of cohort and age. The oldest cohort was born prior to the end of World War II, between 1936 and 1945, and the youngest was born three decades later, between 1966 and 1975.

The cohort differences are large, especially for teenagers and especially relative to the oldest cohort. For example, for those born after World War II, drug use increased by more than a factor of four and dependence given use (susceptibility) also increased by a factor of four or more. Multiplying "use" by "susceptibility" should yield prevalence. By this logic, addiction increased sixteenfold for teenagers born between 1946 and 1955 and as much as fiftyfold for teenagers born between 1966 and 1975. The magnitudes are interesting. They suggest that historical factors may be among the most important determinants of addiction.

First-Person Accounts of Addiction

There is a very interesting literature on the addict's experience of drug use and dependence. These writings include autobiographical pieces (e.g. Burroughs 1961) and ethnographic surveys that rely heavily on interviews with addicts (e.g. Courtwright, Joseph, and Des Jerlais 1989; Waldorf 1983). Many of these narratives follow a pattern that can be briefly stated, and the sequence of events, as told by those addicted, sheds light on the question of whether addicts can choose to stop using drugs.

In most cases, drug use begins in the teen years because it is "cool" and fun. There is an initial honeymoon period when aversive consequences are not apparent. This is followed by addiction (withdrawal symptoms and/or a shift in priorities with drug use becoming increasingly important) and feelings of regret in regard to how much time and money are being spent on drugs. Next comes a relatively long period during which health and welfare gradually decline. During this

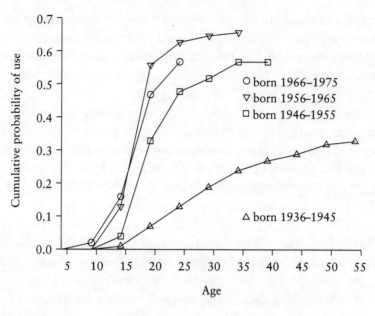

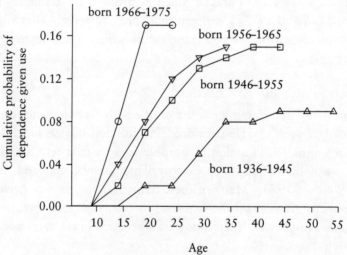

Figure 3.7.   Drug use and dependence given use in men, by age and birth cohort. Source: NCS data, Warner et al. 1995.

period many addicts try to quit, but then relapse after brief periods of abstinence. However, the downward slide usually comes to an end (see recovery rates at beginning of this chapter), and often the end comes in the form of a dramatic realization that life has become intolerable. This realization is often accompanied by intense feelings of shame ("hitting bottom"), reframing of options (for example, "I do not want my kids to think of me as an addict"), and a conscious decision to stop using. Shame and reframing choices do not necessarily lead to changes in drug use, but this occurs often enough for "hitting bottom" to have become a widely recognized turning point in stories of addiction.

Recovery is not simply refraining from drug use. Success typically requires proactive measures, such as avoiding settings and friends associated with drug use and taking up new activities that can replace drug use (hobbies, new love relationships, exercise, and so on). In the initial stages of abstinence, the ex-user may suffer withdrawal symptoms and knows that "just one more hit" will significantly improve things. Moreover, abstinence increases the immediate, rewarding effects of the drug (because tolerance has been reversed). Gradually, though, new activities take over, and drug use loses its strong hold over behavior.

Recovering addicts struggle with their own desires, and success entails the ability to turn away from certain pleasure for an uncertain future. One could argue that abstinence following heavy drug use requires more effort and more self-control than refraining from initial use or never trying to stop. However, to call addiction a disease ignores these distinctions and, more generally, it fails to even acknowledge the efforts and accomplishments of those who do quit. In any case, the story of addiction is marked by choice points, inner struggle, and decisions—not by automatic, blind strivings, as implied by the disease model.

If Addiction Is Voluntary, Why Is It Hard to Quit?

Recovery from addiction is probably always a struggle, and for a significant minority it is a protracted battle (e.g. Vaillant 1992). This may appear to support the disease model. That is, if drug use is a matter of choice, why can't addicts simply quit? A detailed answer to this question is provided in a paper that serves as the theoretical counter-part to this chapter (Heyman 1996a). The paper's thesis is that addiction is a kind of evolutionary accident due to the poor fit between the mechanisms that guide choice and the reward structure of addictive drugs.

Addiction as Drug Preference

Experimental research shows that choice is not guided by rational bookkeeping principles, as often assumed in economic theory, but by myopic, psychological principles that reflect partial and distorted information about the competing alternatives (see Ainslie 1975; Herrnstein 1990; Heyman 1982; Heyman and Tanz 1995). Although myopic, these mechanisms are usually adequate, producing near optimal outcomes under normal conditions (e.g. Herrnstein and Prelec 1992; Heyman and Luce 1979). However, addictive drugs have unusual properties that sabotage optimal outcomes. They provide immediate positive effects and little if any satiation. Hence there are no "natural" brakes on consumption. But the delayed outcomes can be quite delete-rious. This combination of properties implies a net loss for decision processes that are biased in favor of the immediate rather than the de-layed value of a commodity. Also, addictive drugs have the pernicious property of undermining the reward value of competing activities (for example, withdrawal symptoms and intoxication do this; see Heyman 1996a, 1996b). This leads to a narrowing of the behavioral repertoire, with drug use crowding out other behaviors. In short, there is a mis-match, of evolutionary origin, between the rewarding properties of addictive drugs and the normal mechanisms of choice. These "book-keeping" problems are compounded when there are also serious med-ical and psychiatric problems to contend with. Thus the nature of the mechanisms guiding choice, the drugs themselves, and the limited re-sources available to many if not most addicts conspire to make recov-ery from addiction a particularly difficult challenge.

This theory provides an alternative to the disease model. It says that addiction is a consequence of the normal mechanisms that guide choice operating in a context that reveals their limits—namely re-wards that provide large up-front positive values in combination with hidden and delayed costs. This account also implies that to survive their own appetites, individuals require culturally transmitted practices that reinforce self-restraint (Prelec and Herrnstein 1991; Heyman 1996b). In turn, this point implies that cultural variation in the value of self-restraint and individual differences in the tendency to weight short- and long-term goals will influence addiction in important ways. Thus, like the disease model, the "evolutionary mismatch model" accounts for failures in self-command, but unlike the disease model, it views addiction as voluntary (which is to say, subject to contingencies).

The behavioral data favor the "evolutionary mismatch" model over the disease model. To be sure, the struggle for self-command is difficult, but the difficulties are ones that are amenable to contingencies. In contrast, the symptoms of diseases such as schizophrenia and Tourette's syndrome have remained largely immune to the influences of insight, reward, and punishment. Put another way, the biological substrates of addiction are more susceptible to environmental influences than are the biological substrates of many if not all other psychiatric syndromes.

Summary and Discussion

This chapter has presented empirical findings relevant to the widely accepted claim that addiction is a "chronic, relapsing disease." The data show that addiction typically remits, that it is the shortest-lasting psychiatric disorder, that it is the disorder most influenced by socially mediated consequences, and that addicts can curtail drug use when it is immediately beneficial to do so.

These conclusions are not inferences but simply a summary of the research findings. Thus the issue is not so much a question of how to interpret the findings, but whether to believe the findings.

Are the Findings Reliable and Valid?

Many of the graphs and statistics are based on interviews, a method subject to a host of obvious biases. The "data" depend on how questions are framed, how subjects are selected, and what the informants can remember and are willing to say about their own behavior. Moreover, the behavior in question is illegal. Thus it is reasonable to have serious doubts about the reliability and validity of the results.

Recall that the interviews were conducted by lay staff, not by professionally certified clinicians. This raises the possibility that as judged by trained clinicians, the diagnoses were wrongly assigned. However, in a study conducted with a clinic population, there was good agreement (Robins et al. 1982). Of the subjects who had been given a diagnosis by a psychiatrist, 75 percent were given the same diagnosis by the lay researchers. Conversely, for those subjects who were not given a diagnosis by the psychiatrist, 94 percent were also not given a diagnosis by the researchers. Some disorders were easier to agree upon than others. For substance abuse and dependence, 85 percent of cases identified by psychiatrists were also identified by the lay researchers.

But these were current or recent clinic patients, while the epidemiological research was conducted primarily with randomly selected individuals from major American metropolitan areas. The clinic subjects might be easier to diagnose and thus give a misleading account of reliability. Accordingly, the ECA researchers ran a second reliability study, this time with subjects selected independently of treatment history (Helzer et al. 1985). The subjects were first interviewed by a researcher, then by a psychiatrist. The median interval was six weeks so that there was time for symptoms to worsen or improve. The overall level of agreement on whether a subject met the criteria for a substance-use disorder was more than 90 percent. Of those identified by the psychiatrists as having a drug-use disorder, two-thirds were similarly identified by the researchers. Of those identified by the psychiatrists as not suffering from drug dependence or abuse, more than 90 percent were also not given a diagnosis by the researchers.

But reliable diagnoses do not guarantee meaningful results. The informants could systematically lie, or, more likely, misrepresent the past when it was inconsistent with their current situation or with what they thought the interviewer wanted to hear.

Truthfulness

The use of illicit drugs is punishable, and many of those who use illicit drugs have a history of committing illegal acts. Thus there are good reasons to suppose that informants would not be truthful about drug use, especially current drug use. This could explain the high remission rates (honesty about the past but not about the present).

In some settings, those who use illegal drugs often deny that they do so. For instance, in several studies pregnant women who tested positive for cocaine typically denied that they were using illegal drugs, including cocaine (Brownsberger 1997). Moreover, they continued to deny drug use even when confronted with positive urine and meconium samples (e.g. Ostrea et al. 1992; Nair, Rothblum, and Hebel 1994). However, the women were concerned that if they admitted to drug use they might lose their medical assistance or even have their children taken away.

The perceived risks for the interviewees in the studies reviewed in this chapter were different. The researchers went to great lengths to assure the informants that their answers would not be turned over to the legal authorities, that their anonymity would be preserved, and that there would be no negative consequences for participating in the interviews. Objective evidence, such as urine samples, indicates that these assurances established a setting in which truthful answers were the norm. In the Vietnam studies (Robins et al. 1980), 97 percent of those who had an official record of narcotic use while in the army reported this to the interviewers. Urine tests on this population, done after the interview, did not reveal higher rates of current use than did self-report. This is significant in that the veterans did not know they were going to be tested, and the interviewer did not know the informant's history. As noted above, there was a similar level of concordance between official records and the interview data in the St. Louis study (Robins and Murphy 1967).

Validity

Although tests indicate that the ECA researchers reliably classified their informants, these tests do not guarantee that the estimates of relapse rates and duration are valid. For instance, there were no independent checks of when a disorder began or ended. Longitudinal studies could provide more certain information, but such data have not been collected. Thus it may be reasonable to assume that the duration and remission data are inherently flawed.

The basic question is whether the behavioral results shown in the various graphs reflect the researchers' methods or the subjects' behavior. If the findings reflect methods, then they should vary across studies; if the findings reflect the nature of addiction, each type of study should tell essentially the same story.

There was, I believe, a considerable degree of consistency across studies. The research on heroin addiction in Vietnam and St. Louis and the two national surveys led to similar estimates of remission rates and duration. The laboratory findings and the first-person narratives told the same story: depending on the consequences, addicts can choose to abstain. There is even a rough quantitative agreement in the various accounts. A minority of the Vietnam veterans (6 percent) sought clinic-based treatment. Their relapse rates (67 percent) were within the range reported in the clinic-based studies. This suggests that the high recovery rates in the Vietnam sample were not unusual, but exactly what would be seen in a prospective study conducted with addicts who do not seek treatment and who became addicted in the United States.

Treatment

The data and theory presented in this chapter indicate that treatment and policy that devalue the benefits of drug use, that serve to create and strengthen activities that can effectively compete with drugs, and that teach addicts to reframe their options in terms of their full costs and benefits will prove effective. The chapters by Sally L. Satel and George E. Vaillant come to similar conclusions in regard to consequences and alternative activities, although they express these ideas somewhat differently.

Although this chapter has emphasized the role of environmental factors and individual differences in recovery, the emphasis on the biological basis of voluntary behavior implies that pharmacological treatments are potentially valuable resources for reducing drug use. The story of methadone provides a useful example.

Methadone pretreatment attenuates the effects of heroin. The rush and subsequent high are greatly diminished, and as a result preference for heroin decreases. However, whether a decrease in heroin's hedonic effects leads to a resolved recovery appears to depend on additional factors. For instance, Dole and Nyswander's (1967) original methadone programs were highly successful, whereas recent reports show that methadone patients frequently test positive for cocaine, alcohol, and other drugs (e.g. Silverman et al. 1996). One possible explanation for the initial high success rates is that the majority of Dole and Nyswander's patients quickly established interests that could compete with heroin. For example, within six months of starting treatment, about 75 percent were employed. Also, Dole and Nyswander excluded subjects who were least likely to develop alternatives to drug use. Possibly other addictive drugs have practical pharmacological antidotes. This research should be pursued, as pharmacological methods are in principle a highly efficient technique for modifying preferences.

This chapter focused on research in which there was an effort to study representative drug users and not just those who were treated in clinics. When addiction is looked at in this way, it is not a chronic disease but a matter of ambivalent drug use. In the short term, the drug is the better option; in the long term, it is not. The implication for treatment and policy is that addicts can be persuaded to stop using drugs. Moreover, as there is a biology of choice, the techniques of persuasion may include pharmacological agents as well as social ones. In sum, addiction is a malleable disorder, and methods for producing change are well within our reach.

References

Preparation of this chapter was supported by a grant from the Russell Sage Foundation.

Ainslie, G. 1975. "Specious Reward: A Behavioral Theory of Impulsiveness and Control." *Psychological Bulletin* 82: 463–496.

American Psychiatric Association (APA). 1980. *Diagnostic and Statistical Manual of Mental Disorders.* 3rd ed. Washington.

———. 1994. *Diagnostic and Statistical Manual of Mental Disorders.* 4th ed. Washington.

Anthony, J. C., and J. E. Helzer. 1991. "Syndromes of Drug Abuse and Dependence." In Robins and Regier 1991, 116–154.

Ball, J. C., J. W. Shaffer, and D. N. Nurco. 1983. "The Day-to-Day Criminality of Heroin Addicts in Baltimore: A Study in the Continuity of Offense Rates." *Drug and Alcohol Dependence* 12: 119–142.

Biernacki, P. 1986. *Pathways from Heroin Addiction: Recovery without Treatment.* Philadelphia: Temple University Press.

Bigelow, B., and I. Liebson. 1972. "Cost Factors Controlling Alcoholic Drinking." *Psychological Record* 22: 305–314.

Bloom, F. 1997. "The Science of Substance Abuse." *Science* 278: 15.

Brecher, E. 1972. *Licit and Illicit Drugs.* Boston: Little, Brown.

Brown, R., and R. J. Herrnstein. 1975. *Psychology.* Boston: Little, Brown.

Brownsberger, William N. 1997. "Prevalence of Frequent Cocaine Use in Urban Poverty Areas." *Contemporary Drug Problems* 24: 349–371.

Burroughs, W. S. 1961. "Master Addict to Dangerous Drugs." In D. Ebin, ed., *The Drug Experience* (New York: Grove Press), 207–213.

Carroll, Kathleen M., and Bruce J. Rounsaville. 1992. "Contrast of Treatment-Seeking and Untreated Cocaine Abusers." *Archives of General Psychiatry* 49: 464–471.

Chitwood, D. D., and J. S. Chitwood. 1981. "Treatment Program Clients and Emergency Room Patients: A Comparison of Drug-Using Samples." *Journal of Drug Issues* 13: 207–217.

Cohen, M., I. Liebson, L. Faillace, and W. Speers. 1971. "Alcoholism: Controlled Drinking and Incentives for Abstinence." *Psychological Reports* 28: 575–580.

Courtwright, D. T., H. Joseph, and D. Des Jerlais. 1989. *Addicts Who Survived.* Knoxville: University of Tennessee Press.

Dole, V., and M. Nyswander. 1967. "Heroin Addiction: A Metabolic Disease." *Archives of Internal Medicine* 120: 19–24.

Goleman, D. 1990. "How Viewers Grow Addicted to Television." *New York Times,* Oct. 16, C1, C8.

Graeven, D., and K. Graeven. 1983. "Treated and Untreated Addicts: Factors Associated with Participation in Treatment and Cessation of Heroin Use." *Journal of Drug Issues* 13: 207–217.

Helzer, J. E., L. N. Robins, L. T. McEvoy, E. L. Spitzagel, R. K. Stolzman, A. Farmer, and I. F. Brockington. 1985. "A Comparison of Clinical and Diagnostic Interview Schedule Diagnoses." *Archives of General Psychiatry* 42: 657–666.

Helzer, J. E., E. L. Spitzagel, and L. T. McEvoy. 1987. "The Predictive Validity of Lay Diagnoses in the General Population." *Archives of General Psychiatry* 44: 1069–74.

Herrnstein, R. J. 1990. "Behavior, Reinforcement, and Utility." *Psychological Science* 1: 217–224.

Herrnstein, R. J., and D. Prelec. 1992. "A Theory of Addiction." In G. Loewenstein and J. Elster, eds., *Choice over Time* (New York: Russell Sage Foundation), 331–360.

Heyman, G. M. 1982. "Is Time Allocation Elicited Behavior?" In M. Commons, R. J. Herrnstein, and H. Rachlin, eds., *Quantitative Analyses of Behavior,* vol. 2: *Matching and Maximizing Accounts* (Cambridge, Mass.: Ballinger), 459–490.

————. 1996a. "Resolving the Contradictions of Addiction." *Behavioral and Brain Sciences* 19: 561–574.

————. 1996b. "Author's Response." *Behavioral and Brain Sciences* 19: 599–610.

Heyman, G. M., and R. D. Luce. 1979. "Operant Matching Is Not a Logical Consequence of Reinforcement Rate Maximization." *Animal Learning and Behavior* 7: 133–140.

Heyman, G. M., and L. E. Tanz. 1995. "How to Teach a Pigeon to Maximize Overall Reinforcement Rate." *Journal of the Experimental Analysis of Behavior* 64: 277–297.

Hunt, W. A., L. Barnett, and L. Branch. 1971. "Relapse Rates in Addiction Programs." *Journal of Clinical Psychology* 27: 455–456.

Jellinek, E. M. 1960. *The Disease Concept of Alcoholism.* New Haven: Hillhouse Press.

Kessler, R. C., K. A. McGonagle, S. Zhao, C. B. Nelson, M. Hughes, S. Eshleman, H. Wittchen, and K. Kendler. 1994. "Lifetime and 12-Month Prevalence of DSM-III-R Psychiatric Disorders in the United States." *Archives of General Psychiatry* 51: 8–19.

Khantzian, E. 1985. "The Self-Medication Hypothesis of Addictive Disorders: Focus on Heroin and Cocaine Dependence." *American Journal of Psychiatry* 142: 1259–64.

Leshner, A. I. 1997. "Addiction Is a Brain Disease, and It Matters." *Science* 278: 45–47.

Lewis, D. C. 1991. "Comparison of Alcoholism and Other Medical Diseases: An Internist's View." *Psychiatric Annals* 21: 256–265.

Maltzman, I. 1994. "Why Alcoholism Is a Disease." *Journal of Psychoactive Drugs* 26: 13–31.

Miczek, K. 1999. "Aggressive Episodes Impact on Amines and Gene Expression." Master Lecture, 107th Annual Convention of the American Psychological Association, Boston.

Miller, N., and J. Chappel. 1991. "History of the Disease Concept." *Psychiatric Annals* 21: 196–205.

Montoya, I., C. Haertzen, J. Hess, and L. Covi. 1995. "Comparison of Psychological Symptoms between Drug Abusers Seeking and Not Seeking Treatment." *Journal of Nervous and Mental Disease* 183: 50–53.

Nair, P., S. Rothblum, and R. Hebel. 1994. "Neonatal Outcome in Evidence of Fetal Exposure to Opiates, Cocaine, and Cannobinoids." *Clinical Pediatrics* 33: 280–285.

Nash, M. 1997. "The Chemistry of Addiction." *Time,* May 5, 68–76.

Ostrea, E., M. Brady, S. Gause, A. Raymundo, and M. Stevens. 1992. "Drug Screening of Newborns by Meconium Analysis: A Large-Scale, Prospective, Epidemiological Study." *Pediatrics* 89: 107–113.

Prelec, D., and R. J. Herrnstein. 1991. "Preferences or Principles: Alternative Guidelines for Choice." In R. J. Zeckhauser, ed., *Strategy and Choice* (Cambridge, Mass.: MIT Press), 319–340.

Rachlin, H. 1970. *Introduction to Modern Behaviorism.* San Francisco: Freeman.

Regier, D. A., M. E. Farmer, D. S. Rae, B. Z. Locke, S. J. Keith, L. L. Judd, and F. K. Goodwin. 1990. "Comorbidity of Mental Disorders with Alcohol and Other Drug Abuse." *Journal of the American Medical Association* 264: 2511–18.

Regier, D. A., J. K. Myers, M. Kramer, L. N. Robins, D. G. Blazer, R. L. Hough, W. W. Eaton, and B. Z. Locke. 1984. "The NIMH Epidemiological Catchment Area Program." *Archives of General Psychiatry* 41: 934–941.

Robins, L. N. 1993. "Vietnam Veterans' Rapid Recovery from Heroin Addiction: A Fluke or Normal Expectation?" *Addiction* 188: 1041–54.

Robins, L. N., J. E. Helzer, and D. H. Davis. 1975. "Narcotic Use in Southeast Asia and Afterward." *Archives of General Psychiatry* 32: 955–961.

Robins, L., J. E. Helzer, M. Hesselbrock, and E. Wish. 1980. "Vietnam Veterans Three Years after Vietnam: How Our Study Changed Our View of Heroin." In L. Brill and C. Winnick, eds., *The Yearbook of Substance Use and Abuse,* vol. 2 (New York: Human Sciences Press), 214–230.

Robins, L., J. E. Helzer, K. S. Ratcliff, and W. Seyfried. 1982. "Validity of the Diagnostic Interview Schedule, Version II: DSM-III Diagnoses." *Psychological Medicine* 12: 855–870.

Robins, L. N., and G. Murphy. 1967. "Drug Use in a Normal Population of Young Negro Men." *American Journal of Public Health* 57: 1580–96.

Robins, L. N., and D. Regier. 1991. *Psychiatric Disorders in America.* New York: Free Press.

Rounsaville, B. J., and H. D. Kleber. 1985. "Untreated Opiate Addicts." *Archives of General Psychiatry* 42: 1072–77.

Sandifer, M., A. Hordern, G. Timbury, and L. Green. 1968. "Psychiatric Diagnosis: A Comparative Study in North Carolina, London, and Glasgow." *British Journal of Psychiatry* 114: 1–9.

Schelling, T. C. 1992. "Addictive Drugs: The Cigarette Experience." *Science* 255: 430–433.

Searle, J. R. 1983. *Intentionality: An Essay in the Philosophy of Mind.* Cambridge: Cambridge University Press.

Silverman, K., S. Higgins, R. Brooner, I. Montoya, E. Cone, C. Schuster, and L. Kenzie. 1996. "Sustained Cocaine Abstinence in Methadone Maintenance Patients through Voucher-Based Reinforcement Therapy." *Archives of General Psychiatry* 53: 409–415.

Skinner, B. F. 1938. *The Behavior of Organisms: An Experimental Analysis.* New York: Appleton.

Spitzer, R., and J. Forman. 1979. DSM-III Field Trials: II. Initial Experience with the Multiaxial System. *American Journal of Psychiatry* 136: 818–820.

Spitzer, R., J. Forman, and J. Nee. 1979. "DSM-III Field Trial: I. Initial Inter-rater Diagnostic Reliability." *American Journal of Psychiatry* 136: 815–817.

Stephens, R., and E. A. Cottrell. 1972. "A Follow-up Study of 200 Narcotic Addicts Committed for Treatment under the Narcotic Addiction Reha-bilitation Act (NARA)." *British Journal of Addiction* 67: 45–53.

Thombs, D. L. 1994. *Introduction to Addictive Behaviors*. New York: Guil-ford.

Vaillant, G. E. 1966. "Twelve-Year Follow-up of New York Addicts." *American Journal of Psychiatry* 122: 727–737.

———. 1992. "Is There a Natural History of Addiction?" In C. P. O'Brien and J. H. Jaffe, eds., *Addictive States* (New York: Raven Press), 41–57.

Vuchinich, R. 1996. "Addiction as Choice? Yes. As Melioration? Maybe, Maybe Not." *Behavioral and Brain Sciences* 19: 597–598.

Waldorf, D. 1983. "Natural Recovery from Opiate Addiction: Some Social-Psychological Processes of Untreated Recovery." *Journal of Drug Issues* 13: 239–279.

Waldorf, D., C. Reinarman, and S. Murphy. 1991. *Cocaine Changes*. Philadelphia: Temple University Press.

Warner, L., R. C. Kessler, M. Hughes, J. C. Anthony, and C. B. Nelson. 1995. "Prevalence and Correlates of Drug Use and Dependence in the United States." *Archives of General Psychiatry* 52: 219–229.

Wasserman, D. A., M. G. Weinstein, B. E. Havassy, and S. M. Hall. 1998. "Factors Associated with Lapses to Heroin Use during Methadone Maintenance." *Drug and Alcohol Dependence* 52: 183–192.

Wilson, J. Q., and R. J. Herrnstein. 1985. *Crime and Human Nature*. New York: Simon and Schuster.

Wise, R. A., and M. A. Bozarth. 1987. *Psychological Review* 94: 469–492.

Zinberg, N. E., W. M. Harding, and M. A. Winkeller. 1977. "A Study of the Social Regulatory Mechanisms in Controlled Illicit Drug Use." *Journal of Drug Issues* 7: 117–133.

Is Drug Addiction a Brain Disease?

4

Sally L. Satel

More than one hundred substance-abuse experts gathered in Chantilly, Virginia, in November 1995, for a meeting called by the government's top research agency on drug abuse. A major topic was whether the agency, the National Institute on Drug Abuse (NIDA), which is part of the National Institutes of Health, should declare drug addiction a disease of the brain. The experts—academics, public health workers, state officials, and others—said yes, overwhelmingly.

At the time that answer was controversial, but since then the notion of addiction as a brain disease has become widespread, thanks in large measure to a full-blown public-education campaign by NIDA. Waged in editorial boardrooms, town hall gatherings, and Capitol Hill briefings and hearings, the campaign reached its climax in the spring of 1998 when the media personality Bill Moyers catapulted the brain-disease concept into millions of living rooms with his five-part television special. Using imaging technology, Moyers showed viewers eye-catching pictures of addicts' brains under PET scan.[1] The cocaine-damaged parts of the brain were "lit up"—an "image of desire," one researcher called it.

Dramatic visuals are seductive and lend scientific credibility to NIDA's position, but politicians should resist this medicalized portrait for at least two reasons. First, it appears to reduce a complex human activity to a slice of damaged brain tissue. Second, and more important, it vastly underplays the reality that much of addictive behavior is voluntary.

118

The idea of a "no-fault" disease did not originate at NIDA. For the last decade or so it has been vigorously promoted by mental-health advocates working to transform the public's understanding of severe mental illness. Until the early 1980s, remnants of the psychiatric profession and much of the public were still inclined to blame parents for their children's serious mental problems. Then accumulating neuroscientific discoveries began to show, irrefutably, that schizophrenia was marked by measurable abnormalities of brain structure and function. Diseases like schizophrenia and manic-depressive illness were products of a defective brain, not bad parenting.

The mental health movement has drawn momentum from the 20-year-old National Alliance for the Mentally Ill (NAMI), the nation's largest grassroots advocacy organization for people with severe psychiatric disorders and their families. NAMI has mounted a vigorous anti-stigma campaign—slogan: mental illnesses are brain diseases—that has sought to capture public attention through television exposure, publicized opinion polls and surveys, star-studded fundraisers, and frequent congressional testimony. Its success can be seen in the increasing media coverage of severe mental illness, sympathetic made-for-TV specials about the mentally ill, and the widespread assumption, usually explicitly stated by reporters, that these conditions have a biological origin.

While some of those experts who met in Chantilly would say that emphasizing the role of will, or choice, is just an excuse to criminalize addiction, the experience of actually treating addicts suggests that such an orientation provides grounds for therapeutic optimism. It means that the addict is capable of self-control—a much more encouraging conclusion than one could ever draw from a brain-bound, involuntary model of addiction.

The brain-disease model leads us down a narrow clinical path. Since it implies that addicts cannot stop using drugs until their brain chemistry is back to normal, it overemphasizes the value of pharmaceutical intervention. At the same time, because the model also says that addiction is a "chronic and relapsing" condition, it diverts attention from truly promising behavioral therapies that challenge the inevitability of relapse by holding patients accountable for their choices.

Getting a purchase on the true nature of addiction is difficult. Even the definition is elusive. For example, addiction can be defined by pathological state (as a brain disease if affected neurons are examined); by "cure" (as a spiritual disease if vanquished through religious conversion); or by psychodynamics (as a matter of voluntary behavior if addicts are given incentives that successfully shape their actions). Yet when clinicians, scientists, and policymakers are confronted by such definitional choices, it makes the most sense to settle on the one with the greatest clinical utility. In what follows, therefore, I will argue the virtues of thinking about addiction as a primary, though modifiable, behavioral phenomenon, rather than simply as a brain disease. That is, addiction is a function of a person, rather than simply a physical state.

What Does "Brain Disease" Mean?

An NIDA article entitled "Addiction Is a Brain Disease, and It Matters," published in October 1997 in the prestigious journal *Science,* summarizes the evidence that long-term exposure to drugs produces addiction—that is, the compulsion to take drugs—by eliciting changes in specific neurons in the central nervous system. Because these changes are presumed to be irreversible, the addict is perpetually at risk for relapse. The article states:

> Virtually all drugs of abuse have common effects, either directly or indirectly, on a single pathway deep within the brain. Activation of this pathway [the mesolimbic reward system] appears to be a common element in what keeps drug users taking drugs . . . The addicted brain is distinctly different from the non-addicted brain, as manifested by changes in metabolic activity, receptor availability, gene expression and responsiveness to environmental cues . . . That addiction is tied to changes in brain structure and function is what makes it, fundamentally, a brain disease.[2]

The psychiatrist and molecular biologist Steven Hyman puts the biology in a larger, evolutionary context. "Adaptive emotional circuits make brains vulnerable to drug addiction," he says, "because certain addictive drugs mimic or enhance the actions of neurotransmitters used by those circuits."[3] By the time drugs and alcohol have become objects of intense desire, Hyman's research suggests, they've commandeered key motivational circuits away from normal human pleasures, like sex and eating. On a cellular level, bombardment by drugs and alcohol produces chronic adaptations in the neurons of the key circuits, leading to dependence, a state in which the brain "demands" that the addict get high. This is a distinctly different understanding of disease from that promoted by Alcoholics Anonymous, the institution most responsible for popularizing the disease concept of addiction. In AA, disease is employed as a metaphor for loss of control. Thus members might say, "I am unable to drink or take drugs because I have a disease that leads me to lose control when I do." And even though AA assumes that the inability to stop drinking once started is biologically driven, it does not allow this to overshadow its central belief that addiction is a symptom of a spiritual defect. The goal is sobriety through personal growth and the practice of honesty and humility.

The brain-disease advocates are operating in an entirely different frame of reference. Within it they have stipulated that "addiction" means compulsive drug-taking driven by drug-induced brain changes. They assume a correlation between drug-taking behavior and PET scan appearance, though such a correlation has yet to be clearly demonstrated (see note 1), and they speculate, on the basis of preliminary evidence, that subtle changes persist for years. The assumption seems to be that the neuroscience of addiction will give rise to pharmaceutical remedies. But to date the search for a cocaine medication has come up empty. And the disposition to use drugs commonly persists among heroin addicts even after treatment with the best medication for normalizing the compulsion for heroin—methadone. That is because methadone does not, cannot, assuage the underlying anguish for which drugs like heroin and cocaine are the desperate remedy.

A *Time* magazine article entitled "Addiction: How We Get Hooked" asked: "Why do some people fall so easily into the thrall of alcohol, cocaine, nicotine and other addictive substances?" The answer, it said, "may be simpler than anyone dared imagine": dopamine, "the master molecule of addiction ... As scientists learn more about how dopamine works, the evidence suggests that we may be fighting the wrong battle [in the war on drugs]." Among the persons quoted is Nora Volkow, a PET expert at Brookhaven Laboratories, who says, "Addiction . . . is a disorder of the brain no different from other forms of mental illness." That new insight, *Time* intones, may be the "most important contribution" of the dopamine hypothesis to the fight against drugs.[4]

Given the exclusive biological slant and naive enthusiasm of the *Time* article, one is not surprised at its omission of an established fact of enormous clinical relevance: that the course of addictive behavior can be influenced by the very consequences of the drug-taking itself. When the addict reacts to adverse consequences of drug use—economic, health, legal, and personal—by eventually quitting drugs, reducing use, changing his pattern of use, or getting help, he does so voluntarily. Rather than being the inevitable, involuntary product of a diseased brain, these actions represent the essence of voluntariness. The addict's behavior can be modified by knowledge of the consequences.[5] Involuntary behavior cannot.

Clinical Features of Addiction

Addiction as a term does not exist in the formal medical lexicon, but drug addiction is generally equated with "drug dependence." In the American Psychiatric Association's *Diagnostic and Statistical Disorders Manual* (fourth edition), dependence denotes the persistent, compulsive, time-consuming use of a substance despite harmful consequences and often despite an expressed desire not to use it. Most dependent users develop tolerance—they must keep increasing doses to achieve a desired effect. They experience withdrawal symptoms and intense craving when the substance is stopped abruptly, followed by relief when use is resumed.

It is common for heroin-dependent persons to lose the ability to feel euphoric from the drug, yet continue to seek it solely to keep from going into withdrawal ("getting sick"). Withdrawal from heroin (and other opiate drugs including Demerol, morphine, Percocet, and codeine) or from alcohol, but not from cocaine, causes a predictable pattern of physical symptoms. Recall Jack Lemmon in the movie *Days of Wine and Roses,* sweating, anxious, his body racked with tremors, desperate for alcohol after running out of whiskey. Or Frank Sinatra in *Man With the Golden Arm,* the heroin addict suffering painful muscle cramps and powerful cravings for heroin after his last fix wears off.

Unlike heroin and alcohol, cocaine does not produce such physical withdrawal symptoms. The heavy cocaine addict typically uses the drug (by inhalation or injection) in a driven, repetitive manner for 24 to 72 hours straight. Cocaine wears off very quickly, and as it fades the yearning for more is overpowering. Each fresh hit quells the intense craving. The process winds down when the addict becomes too exhausted, runs out of money, or becomes too paranoid, a potential effect of cocaine and other stimulants, such as methamphetamine. He then "crashes" into a phase of agitated depression and hunger, followed by sleep for 12 to 36 hours. Within hours to days after awakening he experiences powerful urges to use, and the cycle resumes.

It is almost impossible for a regular user in the midst of a cocaine binge or experiencing the withdrawal of heroin to stop using the drugs if they are available. He is presumably in the "brain disease" state, when use is most compulsive, neuronal disruption most intense. True, purposeful behavior can occur even in this state—for example, the attempt, sometimes violent, to get money or drugs is highly goal-directed—but at the same time the phase can be so urgent and impossible to derail that addicts ignore their screaming babies, frantically gouge themselves with dirty needles, and ruin families, careers, and reputations.

Nonetheless, most addicts have broken the cycle many times. Either they decide to go "cold turkey" or they end up doing so, unintentionally, by running out of drugs or money or landing in jail. Some heroin addicts admit themselves to the hospital to detoxify because they want to quit; others do so to reduce the cost of their habit, knowing they'll be more sensitive to the effects of heroin afterward. The latter behavior, while motivated by an effort to use drugs more efficiently, is nonetheless a purposeful step that the addict could have taken to reexert lasting control.

In the days between binges cocaine addicts make many deliberate choices, and one of those choices could be the choice to stop using the drug. Heroin-dependent individuals, by comparison, use the drug several times a day but can be quite functional in all respects as long as they have stable access to some form of opiate drug in order to prevent withdrawal symptoms. Certainly some addicts may "nod off" in abandoned buildings, true to stereotype, if they consume more opiate than the amount to which their bodies have developed tolerance, but others can be "actively engaged in activities and relationships," according to the ethnographers Edward Preble and John J. Casey Jr.: "The brief moments of euphoria after each administration constitute a small fraction of their daily lives. The rest of the time they are aggressively pursuing a career . . . hustling."[6]

Not always hustling, however. According to the Office of National Drug Control Policy, as many as 46 percent of drug users not in treatment report legal-only sources of income, and 42 percent report both legal and illegal.[7] The National Institute of Justice found that 33–67 percent of arrested drug users indicate "full and part time work" as their main source of income.[8] These surveys do not relate income source to severity of addiction, and it is reasonable to assume that the heaviest users participate least in the legitimate economy. Nonetheless, the fact that many committed drug users do have jobs shows that addiction does not necessarily preclude deliberate, planned activity.

Interrupting the Addictive Process

In *The Moral Sense* (1993), James Q. Wilson distinguishes between the road to addiction and the state of being an addict. "Addiction is the result of a series of small choices that provide large immediate benefits but much larger and unwanted long-term costs," he writes, "but by the time the costs are fully understood, the user lacks the ability to forgo the drug the next time it becomes available." Indeed, the inability to forgo drug use is the hallmark of the addict's involuntary "brain disease." Nonetheless, the compulsion to take drugs does not dominate an addict's minute-to-minute or day-to-day existence. There are times when he is capable of reflection and purposeful behavior. During a cocaine addict's week there are periods when he is neither engaged in a binge nor racked with intense craving for the drug. Likewise, during the course of a heroin addict's day he may feel calm and his thoughts may be lucid when he is confident of access to the drug and is using it in doses adequate to prevent withdrawal symptoms but not large enough to be sedating. At these times the addict is not the helpless victim of a brain disease.

Recall the Sinatra character Frankie in *Man With the Golden Arm.* In the last scenes of the film, Frankie makes a purposeful, life-transforming move: he asks his girlfriend, played by Kim Novak, to lock him in a room to prevent him from buying more heroin. Imprisoned in a dreary walk-up, he spends a few days writhing miserably on the floor, begging to be released, pleading for a fix; but Novak holds firm, and days later, her man emerges calm and intact. This dramatic scene, while not medically recommended, illustrates how planned action can break the cycle of use. True, Frankie would have been helpless to control himself if not sequestered, but the point is that he made a deliberate effort to deny himself the opportunity. When properly "fixed," the heroin addict might rationally decide to enter a detoxification or methadone-maintenance program. Between binges the cocaine addict could decide to enter a treatment program or move across town, away from visual cues and personal associations that provoke craving. Yes, addicts *could* do these things—that is, no involuntary disease state is governing them—but if asked to do so, would they?

Probably not. Even those who wish passionately for a better life are often kept entrenched by a profound fear of coping with life without drugs or by the despair of believing there is nothing better available for them. But for some the chances of saying no to the drug can depend on what is at stake. Practically speaking, many necessary things heretofore taken for granted could be put at risk if society decided to make them contingent upon abstinence: examples are welfare payments, employment, public housing, child custody.

A systematic plan that closes all avenues of support to those who cannot or will not stop using drugs—allowing them only elective treatment or, once arrested for nonviolent drug-related crime, court-ordered treatment—seems radical. For one thing, it would require that the treatment system, especially costly residential treatment, be greatly expanded. For another, the policy of refusing addicts access to many public goods and services—or, better, administering small punishments or rewards contingent on performance—might strike some as unfair and objectionable.

But such a policy is not unethical according to a behavioral model of addiction. Society can legitimately place expectations and demands on addicts because their "brain disease" is not a persistent state. By contrast, it would be unthinkable to expect "victims" of true involuntary disease to control their afflictions. We would never demand that an epileptic marshal his will power to control a seizure, or that a breast cancer patient stop her tumor from metastasizing. Experimental evidence shows, however, that addicts can control drug-taking. In his book *Heavy Drinking: The Myth of Alcoholism as a Disease,* the philosopher Herbert Fingarette refutes the premise that alcoholism represents an inevitable total loss of control. He cites numerous independent investigations conducted under controlled conditions in behavioral laboratories showing the degree to which alcoholics are capable of regulating themselves. Researchers found, for example, that the amount of alcohol consumed was related to its cost and the effort required to obtain it. Once offered small payments, subjects were able to refuse freely available alcohol. And after they had drunk an initial "priming" dose, the amount they subsequently consumed was inversely proportionate to the size of the payment.

Fingarette acknowledges that these results were obtained with hospitalized alcoholics who were also receiving social support and help. Perhaps, he says, the change in setting from home to hospital radically affects alcoholics' self-control and drinking patterns. Still, this "explanation undermines the classic loss-of-control conjecture . . . It is the social setting, not any chemical effect of alcohol, that influences drinkers' ability to exert control over their drinking." Other experiments have shown that the drinkers' beliefs and attitudes about alcohol influence how much they consume.[9]

The story of the returning Vietnam servicemen is a revealing natural experiment that "changed our views of heroin," according to the epidemiologist Lee Robins and her colleagues, who wrote the now classic paper on the subject.[10] They found that only 14 percent of men who were dependent on heroin in Vietnam—and who failed a publicized urine test at departure—resumed regular heroin use within three years of their return home. The rest had access to heroin and even used some occasionally, but what made them decide to stop for good,

Robins found, was the "sordid" culture surrounding heroin use, the price, and fear of arrest.

"Chronic and Relapsing" Brain Disease?

Given the heavy biomedical orientation at the National Institutes of Health, a phrase like "chronic brain disease" is a device that aligns NIDA's mission with that of its parent. Away from home, the major political purpose of the model is to establish a moral and clinical equivalence between addiction and other medical conditions. Diabetes, asthma, and high blood pressure are the trio most often cited as prototypical "chronic and relapsing" disorders. NIDA predicts that medicalization will destigmatize compulsive drug-taking and shift the commonly held perception of addicts from "bad people" to be dealt with by the criminal justice system to "chronic illness sufferers" to be triaged to medical care. In the words of a recent NIDA report, "Vigorous and effective leadership is needed to inform the public that addiction is a medical disorder . . . [It is not] self-induced or a failure of will."[11]

This is also the agenda of the newly formed group Physician Leadership on National Drug Policy, whose prestigious members include the former president of the AMA, a Nobel Prize winner, leaders at the Department of Health and Human Services, a former FDA director, and the Surgeon General. The result of "concerted efforts to eliminate stigma" should be that substance abuse is "accorded parity with other chronic, relapsing conditions insofar as access to care, treatment benefits and clinical outcomes are concerned," according to a statement from Physician Leadership.[12] These sentiments have been echoed in reports from the Institute of Medicine. "Addiction . . . is not well understood by the public and policymakers. Overcoming problems of stigma and misunderstanding will require educating the public . . . about the progress made," a 1997 report says.[13]

By changing popular opinion, these institutions hope to work through federal and state legislatures to secure more treatment, expanded insurance coverage, and other services for addicts as well as more funding for addiction research. These are not unreasonable aims insofar as substandard quality of care, limited access to care, and understudied research questions remain active problems. But the destigmatizing approach has been too readily borrowed from the mental health community. Along with the obvious deterrent value, stigmatizing is necessary to help enforce societal norms. Furthermore, forcing a rigid barrier between the so-called medical and moral arenas eclipses one of the most promising venues for anti-addiction efforts: the criminal justice system (the courts and probation services), which can impose sanctions that greatly deter relapse.

The *Science* article asserts: "If the brain is the core of the problem, attending to the brain needs to be the core of the solution." How are we to do this? By using either "medications or behavioral treatments to reverse or compensate for brain changes." The idea of medication is indeed a logical one—its effectiveness, to be discussed later, is another matter—and medications can certainly affect the brain. Even behavioral treatments, in the case of obsessive-compulsive illness, have been documented to alter the brain. Indeed, any effective behavioral treatments change the brain; otherwise there would be no lasting cognitive or emotional transformations. But to say that all treatments must work primarily on the brain is misleading. To extend this line of reasoning to recovery through religious conversion, a well-established phenomenon, one would have to say that spirituality first led to a brain change that then enabled the individual to defeat his habit—a bizarre, reductionistic way, it seems, of thinking about the inspirational properties of religion, and one that underscores the impoverished clinical vocabulary of the brain-disease model.

Patients are not passive recipients of "doses" of medicine or therapy; they are participants in a dynamic process that, among other things, requires them to fight their urges to use drugs, discover ways to minimize those urges, and find alternative forms of gratification. This is hard work, and most addicts who volunteer for it do so under duress, compelled by the threat of loss—loss of job, relationships, custody of children, even their own freedom.

In an article in *Lancet* entitled "Myths about the Treatment of Addiction," the researchers Charles P. O'Brien and A. Thomas McLellan state that relapse to drugs is an inherent aspect of addiction and should not be viewed as a treatment failure: "Addiction should be [considered] a brain disease, similar to other chronic and relapsing conditions [in which] considerable improvement is considered successful treatment even though complete remission or cure is not achieved." They argue that (1) relapse in long-term conditions like asthma, diabetes, and hypertension is often due to the patient's poor compliance with prescribed diet, exercise, or medication; (2) an addict's relapse is a result of poor compliance; thus (3) addiction is like other diseases.[14]

But this is reversed. Asthmatics and diabetics who resist their doctors' orders resemble addicts, rather than addicts' resembling them. Asthmatics and diabetics may deteriorate spontaneously for physical reasons that are unprovoked and unavoidable; relapse to addiction, by contrast, invariably represents a failure to comply with "doctors' orders"—that is, to stop using drugs. Similarly confused are comparisons between addiction and medical conditions like cancer, epilepsy, and schizophrenia that were once stigmatized as resulting from personal weakness.[15] In cancer and epilepsy, the tumor and the seizure *result* from abnormal physiological processes, while drug abuse *produces* deranged physiology.

If one looks only at clinic-outcome studies, the claim that addiction is a chronic and relapsing disease has ample support, but data from the large Epidemiologic Catchment Area (ECA) study, funded by the National Institute of Mental Health, show that in the general population, long periods of remission, even permanent remission, for drug dependence (addiction) and drug abuse are the norm, not the exception.[16] According to ECA criteria for remission—defined as no symptoms for the year just prior to the interview—59 percent of roughly 1,300 respondents who met criteria for being users at some point in their lives were at that time free of drug problems. The average duration of remission was 2.7 years, and the mean duration of illness was 6.1 years, with about three-fourths of the cases lasting no more than 8 years. Because the ECA, which surveyed a total of 20,300 adults, did not analyze drug abuse and drug dependence separately, it is impossible to know how the two differed: presumably, dependent users had longer durations of active symptoms and shorter remissions. Even so, these figures suggest that addiction is not an enduring problem in everyone it afflicts.

Drug Cures for Drug Addiction?

The pharmacological imperative is a logical outgrowth of placing the brain at the center of the addictive process. Still, attempts to treat addiction with other drugs or medications have been around for centuries. In the NIDA budget, about 15 percent goes to the Medications Development Division, which was authorized by Congress in 1992. One of NIDA's major goals was the development of an anti-cocaine medication by the turn of the century. But no magic bullet has appeared, and the NIDA director has downgraded predictions about the curative power of medication, promoting it as potentially "complementary" to behavioral therapy.

It is always possible, of course, that an effective drug will be developed. But it is important, for the sake of the public's trust and NIDA's credibility, that the brain-disease advocates not oversell the promise of medications. To date, more than 40 pharmaceuticals have been studied in randomized controlled trials in human beings for their effect on cocaine abuse or dependence. Some of these were intended to block craving, others to substitute for cocaine itself; none has yet proved even minimally effective. The basic problem with the anti-craving medications is their lack of specificity. Instead of deploying a surgical strike on the neuronal site of cocaine yearning, they end up blunting motivation in general and may also depress mood. Experiments with substitution drugs (for example, cocaine-like substances such as methylphenidate) have proven equally frustrating, because instead of suppressing the urge to use, they tend to act like an appetizer, producing physical sensations and emotional memories reminiscent of cocaine itself and consequently triggering a desire for the real thing.[17]

If a selective medication could be developed, it might be especially helpful to cocaine addicts who have been abstinent for a time but who experience a sudden burst of craving for the drug, a feeling that is often reported as alien, coming from "out of nowhere," and different from a true desire to use cocaine. Such a craving may be triggered by some kind of environmental cue, such as passing through the neighborhood where the addict used to get high. Generally, the recovering addict learns his idiosyncratic cues, avoids them, and arms himself with exercises and strategies (such as immediately calling a 12-Step sponsor) that help him fight the urge. It is conceivable that a medication could help suppress the jolt of desire and, ultimately, uncouple the cue from the conditioned response.

Another approach to cocaine addiction is immunization against the drug's effect.[18] In late 1995 scientists reported promising results of tests of a cocaine vaccine in rats. The animals were inoculated with an artificial cocaine-like substance that triggered the production of antibodies to cocaine. When actual cocaine was administered, the antibodies attached themselves to the molecules of cocaine, reducing the amount of free drug available in the bloodstream to enter the brain. Immunized rats showed less cocaine-induced movement and sniffing, and when their brains were examined, the levels of cocaine were 50–80 percent lower than in non-immunized rats.

The vaccine is still being developed for use in humans, but the principle behind its presumed effect—behavioral "extinction"—is already being exploited by an available anti-heroin medication called naltrexone. Naltrexone blocks opiate molecules at the site of attachment to receptors on the neuron. Both naltrexone and the cocaine vaccine create a situation in which an addict who takes the illicit drug will feel little or no effect. Uncoupling the desired response (getting high) from the action intended to produce it (shooting up) is called "extinction," and according to behaviorist theory, the addict will eventually stop using a drug if he no longer achieves an effect. Though naltrexone is technically effective, most heroin addicts reject it in favor of methadone, which gives a mild high and has a calming effect. There are a few groups, however, who will take naltrexone with good results: impaired professionals (such as doctors, lawyers, nurses) who risk loss of their licenses, and probationers and defendants on work release who are closely supervised and urine-tested frequently.

The Methadone Success

Optimism surrounding the pharmaceutical approach to drug dependence stems from the qualified success of methadone, an opiate painkiller that was developed by German chemists during World War II. First tested in 1964 as a substitute for heroin in the United States, methadone is now administered in maintenance clinics to about 19 percent of the nation's estimated 600,000 heroin addicts. Numerous studies have documented the socioeconomic benefits of methadone: significant reductions in crime, overdoses, unemployment, and, in some regions, HIV.[19]

Unlike heroin, which needs to be administered every four to eight hours to prevent withdrawal symptoms, methadone requires a single daily dose. A newly available medication called LAAM (levo-alpha-acetyl-methadol) can prevent withdrawal and craving for up to 72 hours. As a combination substitute and blocker, methadone and its cousin LAAM reduce or obliterate the craving for heroin. In addition, an addict on methadone maintenance who takes heroin will be blocked from experiencing a potent high. Like the drug for which it substitutes, methadone is addictive.

"Successful methadone users are invisible," the director of the Beth Israel Medical Center in New York City told the *New York Times*. Between 5 and 20 percent remain on the medication for over ten years. Jimmie Maxwell, an 80-year-old jazz trumpet player, has stayed clean for the past 32 years by taking methadone every day. "I never missed a day of practice," he told the reporter Christopher Wren. Unfortunately, people who like Maxwell lead a fully productive life and are otherwise drug-free may represent only 5–7 percent of methadone patients.[20] As many as 35–60 percent also use cocaine or other illicit drugs or black-market sedatives.[21] A six-year follow-up of treated addicts found that over half were readmitted to their agency at some point.[22]

This is not surprising. Methadone will only prevent withdrawal symptoms and the related physiological hunger for heroin. To be sure, a heroin addict who is given this opiate is much more likely to stay engaged in a treatment program, but methadone cannot make up for the psychic deficits that led to addiction, such as deep-seated intolerance of boredom, depression, stress, anger, and loneliness. The addict who began heavy drug use in his teens has not even completed the maturational tasks of adolescence; he has not developed social competence, consolidated a personal identity, or formed a concept of his future. Furthermore, methadone cannot solve the secondary layer of troubles that accumulate over years of drug use: family and relationship problems, educational deficiencies, health problems, economic losses. Consequently, only a small fraction of heroin addicts are able to become fully productive on methadone alone.

The failure to recognize this clinical reality was evident at a November 1997 NIH-NIDA conference I attended called "The Medical Treatment of Heroin Addiction." So pervasive was the idea that a dysfunctional brain is the root of addiction that I sat through the entire two-and-a-half-day meeting without once hearing such words as "responsibility," "choice," "character"—the vocabulary of personhood. In fairness, speakers did acknowledge the importance of so-called psychosocial services, but they tended to view these as add-ons, helpful offerings to "keep" patients in the clinic while methadone, the core treatment, did its job. Not unexpectedly, the 12-member panel concluded in its publicized consensus statement that "opiate drug addictions are diseases of the brain . . . that indeed can be effectively treated," and they "strongly recommend[ed] broader access to methadone maintenance treatment programs for people who are addicted to heroin or other opiate drugs."

The Residential Advantage

Unfortunately, the panel overlooked evidence showing that residential treatment is comparable to methadone (perhaps better) from both economic and quality-of-life perspectives. First, enduring benefit from methadone accrues only after the addict spends at least 360 days in the program. According to longitudinal studies, however, only 30–40 percent of an enrolled cohort stays beyond that 360-day point.[23] By comparison, treatment in a residential setting (without methadone) yields benefit after just 90 days, and, similarly, 30–40 percent of that cohort remains enrolled beyond the critical point. Phoenix House residential programs, which represent about 15 percent of the country's residential beds, actually retain 40 percent of their patients at the one-year mark, though most other residential programs continue to engage only about one in ten. Second, as for quality of life, although methadone is obviously less restrictive of patients' freedom than residential treatment, it does place long-term limits on that freedom by tethering patients to rigid dispensing regulations and clinic hours.

Relative to methadone maintenance, an equal or greater proportion of patients in residential treatment participate long enough for the treatment to have a social impact. In fact, in comparing patient outcomes, researchers found that enrollees in methadone maintenance and those in residential treatment had almost identical rates (about 27 percent) of a "highly favorable outcome"—defined as no use of drugs (except, possibly, marijuana) and no arrests or incarcerations within a year after treatment.[24] Likewise, "moderately favorable" results were 41 and 40 percent, respectively. And although the cost of residential treatment is three to five times that of methadone maintenance, the considerable savings in averted crime and resumed productivity associated with residential care, given its much earlier effectiveness (90 days compared to methadone's 360), make its benefit-to-cost ratio more than twice that of methadone maintenance.

Phoenix House Foundation runs the largest network of residential programs in the country. Its philosophy is that the addict himself, not the drug (or his brain), is the primary problem. Thus the rehabilitation seeks to transform the destructive patterns of feeling, thinking, and behaving that make a recovering addict vulnerable to relapse. Group support and self-help are the therapeutic dynamic: residents continually reinforce for one another the expectations and rules of the community. All residents must work, above all so that they learn to accept authority and supervision, abilities vital to future success in the workforce. Residential programs last between 18 and 24 months, "only a fraction of the 21 years it normally takes to raise a person," says the psychiatrist Mitchell Rosenthal, Phoenix House president. Those who complete the program—only one in five do—have an excellent chance of success: five to seven years later 90 percent are still working and law-abiding, and 70 percent are completely drug free.[25] Contrast this to the less-than-one-in-ten rate of methadone-maintained addicts who become fully productive.

Given these outcomes, plus the fact that methadone patients are tied to a medication and the clinic that dispenses it, methadone does not deserve to be the sole beneficiary of the NIDA consensus statement. Residential slots are in gross undersupply—there are only 15,000 nationwide, outnumbered by methadone slots ten to one—and the consensus panel would have done well to call for greater opportunities in that domain as well.

Needed: Enlightened Coercion

"The biggest single need in this country is for a cocaine medication," asserted Alan I. Leshner, the director of NIDA. "We have nothing now other than behavioral treatments."[26] But behavioral therapies make the most practical and theoretical sense. The literature on treatment effectiveness consistently shows that an addict who completes a treatment program—any program—either stops or markedly reduces his use of drugs after discharge. The problem is that only a small number of participants finish their programs. Estimates of attendance beyond 52 weeks, the generally accepted minimum duration for treatment, range from 8 to 20 percent of the patients entering any of the three most common types of programs: outpatient counseling, methadone maintenance, and residential treatment.[27] Clearly, the biggest challenge to any treatment program is keeping patients in it.

How best to instill "motivation" is a perennial topic among clinicians; at least one form of psychotherapy has been developed for that explicit purpose. But routinely neglected by most mainstream addiction experts is the powerful yet counterintuitive fact that patients who enter treatment involuntarily, under court order, fare as well as, and sometimes even better than, those who enroll voluntarily. Numerous studies, including large government-funded studies spanning three decades—the Drug Abuse Reporting Program (1970s), the Treatment Outcome Prospective Study (1980s), and the Drug Abuse Treatment Outcome Study (1990s)—all found that the longer a person stays in treatment, the better his outcome. Not surprisingly, those under legal supervision stay longer than their voluntary counterparts.

Compulsory Residential Treatment

The best-studied population of coerced addicts were part of California's Civil Addict Program (CAP), started in 1962. During its most active years, in the seventies, the program was impressively successful. It required addicts to be treated in a residential setting for two years and then closely supervised by specially trained parole officers for another five. These officers had small caseloads, performed weekly urine tests, and had the authority to return recovering addicts to treatment if they resumed drug use. Most of the addicts had been remanded to CAP for nonviolent drug-related crimes, but some were sent because their addictions were so severe they were unable to care for themselves. Those in the latter group were civilly committed in much the same way that gravely disabled mentally ill persons are often institutionalized.

The success came after a difficult start. During the first 18 months, many California judges, unfamiliar with the new procedures, released patients on a writ of habeas corpus almost immediately after they'd been committed. This judicial blunder, however, allowed Douglas Anglin and his colleagues to conduct an extensive evaluation of nearly 1,000 addicts, comparing those who received compulsory treatment with those who were mistakenly freed.[28] The two groups were otherwise comparable with respect to drug use and demographics. The researchers found that 22 percent of the addicts who were committed reverted to heroin use and crime; this was less than half the rate for the prematurely released group. Other large-scale studies, including the Drug Abuse Reporting Program and the Treatment Outcome Prospective Study, convincingly show, as a result of compulsory treatment, a sustained rate of reduction in drug use and criminal behavior similar to or better than the reduction achieved by voluntary patients.

Though still legally on the books, the Civil Addict Program has become moribund, but the practice of court-ordered residential treatment continues. Unfortunately, parole and probation officers today are not nearly as scrupulous in supervising their charges as were their CAP counterparts. Among the exceptions is a program developed by the Brooklyn, New York, district attorney called Drug Treatment Alternative to Prison (DTAP). It is the first prosecution-run program in the country to divert prison-bound drug offenders to residential treatment. The program targets drug-addicted felons with prior nonviolent convictions who have been arrested for sales to undercover agents. Offenders have their prosecution deferred if they enter the 15-to-24-month program, and their charges are dismissed if they successfully complete the program. DTAP's one-year retention rate of 57 percent is markedly superior to the 13–25 percent rate typically seen in residential treatment. Recidivism to crime at 6, 12, and 24 months after program completion is consistently half that of DTAP-eligible defendants who were regularly prosecuted and sent to prison.[29]

Drug Courts: Treatment and Sanctions

In addition to coercing criminally involved addicts into residential treatment, the criminal justice system is in an excellent position to use sanctions as leverage for compliance with outpatient treatment. Since 1989 it has been doing so through "drug courts," specialized courts that offer nonviolent defendants the possibility of a dismissed charge if they plead guilty and agree to be diverted to a heavily monitored drug treatment program overseen by the drug-court judge. During regularly scheduled status hearings, the judge holds the defendant publicly accountable for his progress by taking into account dirty or missed urine tests and cooperation with the treatment program. Successes are rewarded, and violations are penalized immediately, though in a graduated fashion, starting with small impositions. Repeated failure generally results in incarceration.

Early data on more than 80 drug courts show an *average* retention rate (defined as the sum of all participants who either have completed or are still in drug-court programs) of 71 percent. Even the *lowest* rate of 31 percent greatly exceeds the average one-year retention rate of about 10–15 percent for noncriminal addicts in public-sector treatment programs.

One study conducted by the Urban Institute was designed to examine the influence of sanctions on offenders in the District of Columbia drug court.[30] Three options were followed: (1) the "sanctions track"—urines were obtained twice weekly, and there were increasingly severe penalties (such as a day or more in jail) for missed or dirty urines; (2) the "treatment track"—intensive treatment for several hours a day, without predictable sanctions for missed or dirty urines; (3) the control group—urine tests twice a week, but without predictable sanctions. Researchers found that treatment-track participants were twice as likely to be drug-free in the month before sentencing as those in the control group (27 vs. 12 percent), while sanctions-track participants were three times as likely to be drug-free (37 vs. 12 percent). The certainty of consequences was psychologically powerful to the participants. The researcher Adele Harrell learned in her focus groups with study participants that they credited their ability to stay clean to the "swiftness of the penalties—they had to report to court immediately for a test failure—and their fairness."

And the longer participants stayed in drug court, the better they fared. According to information maintained by the Drug Court Clearinghouse at American University, the differences in rearrest rates were significant. Drug courts operational for 18 months or more reported a completion rate of 48 percent. Depending upon the characteristics and degree of social dysfunction of the graduates, the rate of rearrest—for drug crimes, primarily—within one year of graduation was 4 percent. Even among those who never finished the program (about one in three fail to complete it), rearrest one year after enrollment ranged from 5 to 28 percent. Contrast this with the 26–40 percent one-year rearrest rate reported by the Bureau of Justice Statistics for traditionally adjudicated individuals convicted of drug possession.[31]

These examples show how law enforcement brings addicts into a treatment system, enhances the probability that they will stay, and imposes sanctions for poor compliance with treatment. (The Urban Institute study even forces one to question whether treatment is invariably necessary, since the sanctions-without-treatment track had considerably better results than the treatment-without-sanctions tract.) They also highlight the folly of dividing addicts into two camps: "bad people" for the criminal justice system to dispose of, and "chronic-illness sufferers" for medical professionals to treat. If the brain-disease model transforms every addict into a "sufferer," then the use of coercion to change that person's behavior seems impossible to justify. Thus the brain-disease model fails to accommodate one of the most productive approaches in the history of anti-drug efforts.

Entitlements as Shapers of Behavior

The perception of the addict as a "chronic illness sufferer" also diverts attention from another very promising approach: the use of public entitlements to shape behavior. The Veterans Administration is conducting two demonstration projects wherein addicted, mentally ill veterans "turn over" their sizable monthly benefits to a payee who manages their money and distributes it as a reward contingent upon compliance with treatment. Compare this so-called contingency management to the now defunct federal disability program for addicts, Supplemental Security Income's "DA&A" program. From 1972 to 1994, poor addicts were eligible for income maintenance and federal benefits solely because they had the medical disability of addiction. Not surprisingly, cash often went to purchase drugs, designated payees were sometimes addicts themselves, and few recipients attended treatment. According to the Department of Health and Human Services, less than 1 percent of a cohort of recipients followed for four years left the rolls through "recovery."[32]

A large body of research shows that contingency management (CM) of the sort the Veterans Administration is trying can be successfully applied. One of the earliest studies involved deteriorated, skidrow alcoholic volunteers. Ten were randomly chosen to be eligible for housing, medical care, clothing, and employment services if their blood alcohol levels were below a minimum level. The other ten could obtain these services from the Salvation Army as usual. The volunteers who were rewarded for not drinking did far better at maintaining sobriety and employment.[33]

More recent controlled research on CM uses vouchers redeemable for goods. Much of it has been conducted by the psychologists Steve Higgins and Kenneth Silverman, whose work consistently demonstrates that cocaine and heroin abusers substantially reduce or cease drug use and remain in treatment longer when they are given goods-redeemable vouchers for each negative urine submitted. Silverman and colleagues also conducted a small pilot project in which unemployed heroin users on methadone significantly increased their attendance at job-skills training when they were given vouchers based on attendance.[34]

The contingency-management model has implications for other forms of public largesse, including welfare. About 20–25 percent of mothers on welfare or TANF (Temporary Aid to Needy Families) are estimated to abuse drugs, and many states are considering a treatment requirement for these recipients.[35] But since dropout rates from treatment are high, simply prescribing treatment-as-usual for these women may not reduce their drug use to the point of employability.

Welfare reform provides an excellent opportunity to transform the perverse reward of public entitlements into constructive incentives that promote recovery and autonomy by using the very same benefits that the system now offers. In this way, states could capitalize on the proven virtues of leverage to enhance retention in treatment and to shape behavior directly.

Concluding Observations

Labeling addiction a chronic and relapsing brain disease succeeds more as sloganism than as public health education. By locating addiction in the brain, not the person, NIDA has generated an unwarranted level of enthusiasm about pharmacology for drug addiction. By downplaying the volitional dimension of addiction, the brain-disease model detracts from the great promise of strategies and therapies that rely on sanctions and rewards to shape self-control. And by reinforcing a dichotomy between punitive and clinical approaches to addiction, the model devalues the enormous contribution of criminal justice to combating addiction.

The fact that many, perhaps most, addicts are in control of their actions and appetites for circumscribed periods of time shows that they are not perpetually helpless victims of a chronic disease. They are instigators of their addiction, just as they are agents of their own recovery . . . or nonrecovery. The potential for self-control should allow society to endorse expectations and demands of addicts that would never be made of someone with a true involuntary illness. Making such demands is, of course, no assurance that they'll be met. But confidence in their very legitimacy would encourage a range of policy and therapeutic options—using consequences and coercion—that is incompatible with the idea of a no-fault brain disease.

Efforts to neutralize the stigma of addiction by convincing the public that the addict has a "brain disease" are understandable, but in the long run they have no more likelihood of success than the use of feel-good slogans to help a child acquire "self-esteem." Neither respectability nor a sense of self-worth can be bestowed; both must be earned. The best way for any institution, politician, or advocate to combat the stigma of addiction is to promote conditions—both within treatment settings and in society at large—that help the addict develop self-discipline and, along with it, self-respect. In this way, former addicts become visible symbols of hard work, responsibility, and lawfulness—potent antidotes to stigma.

This prescription does not deny whatever biological or psychological vulnerabilities individuals may have. Instead, it makes their struggle to master themselves all the more ennobling.

Notes

1. Positron emission tomography (PET) allows researchers to visualize brain metabolic function. Using radioactively labeled glucose or other compounds tailored to specific types of cellular receptors (such as the dopamine receptor), researchers can create brain maps by measuring the levels of metabolism or receptor activity in particular brain regions. For example, PET scans of cocaine addicts obtained at two weeks, one month, and four months after last use show persistent decrements in dopamine metabolism. N. D. Volkow et al., "Changes in Brain Glucose Metabolism in Cocaine Dependence and Withdrawal," *American Journal of Psychology* 148 (1991): 621–626. Despite a virtual library of documented, replicable brain changes with drug exposure (in receptor activity, intracellular biochemical changes, blood flow, glucose metabolism, and more), there have been no scientific studies correlating them with behavior, according to the biochemist Bertha Madras of Harvard Medical School.
2. A. I. Leshner, "Addiction Is a Brain Disease, and It Matters," *Science* 278 (1997): 45–47.
3. Institute of Medicine, *Dispelling the Myths about Addiction* (Washington: National Academy of Sciences Press, 1997), 44–46.
4. "Addiction: How We Get Hooked," *Time,* May 5, 1997.
5. See G. M. Heyman, "Resolving the Contradictions of Addiction," *Behavioral and Brain Science* 19 (1996): 561–610.
6. Edward Preble and John J. Casey Jr., "Taking Care of Business: The Heroin User's Life on the Street," in D. E. Smith and G. R. Gay, eds., *It's So Good, Don't Even Try It Once: Heroin in Perspective* (Englewood Cliffs, N.J.: Prentice Hall, 1972), ch. 7.
7. Office of National Drug Control Policy, "Reducing Drug Abuse in America," Feb. 1997.
8. U.S. Dept. of Justice, Office of Justice Programs, "Crack, Cocaine Powder and Heroin: Drug Use and Purchasing Patterns in Six U.S. Cities," Research Report, Nov. 1997.

9. H. Fingarette, *Heavy Drinking: The Myth of Alcoholism as a Disease* (Berkeley: University of California Press, 1989), 37. B. Bigelow and I. Liebson, "Cost Factors Controlling Alcoholic Drinking," *Psychological Record* 22 (1972): 305–314; T. F. Barbor et al., "Experimental Analysis of the 'Happy Hour': Effects of Purchase Price on Alcohol Consumption," *Psychopharmacology* 58 (1978): 35–41.

10. L. N. Robins et al., "Vietnam Veterans Three Years after Vietnam: How Our Study Changed Our Views of Heroin," in L. Brill and C. Winick, eds., *Yearbook of Substance Use and Abuse*, vol. 2 (New York: Human Science Press, 1980).

11. National Institutes of Health, "Effective Medical Treatment of Heroin Addiction," Consensus Development Statement, rev. draft, Nov. 19, 1997, p. 9.

12. Physician Leadership on National Drug Policy, Consensus Statement, July 9, 1997. See also "Medical News and Perspective," *Journal of American Medical Association* 278, no. 5 (1997): 378.

13. Institute of Medicine, *Dispelling the Myths*, 1.

14. C. P. O'Brien and A. T. McLellan, "Myths about the Treatment of Addiction," *Lancet* 347 (1996): 237–240.

15. Institute of Medicine, deliberations of the Committee to Identify Strategies to Raise the Profile of Substance Abuse and Alcoholism Research, 1996.

16. James C. Anthony and John E. Helzer, "Syndromes of Drug Abuse and Dependence," in L. N. Robins and D. A. Regier, eds., *Psychiatric Disorders in America: The Epidemiologic Area Catchment Study* (New York: Free Press, 1991), ch. 6.

17. C. P. O'Brien, "A Range of Research-Based Pharmacotherapies for Addiction," *Science* 278 (1997): 66–70.

18. Ibid.

19. Institute of Medicine, *Federal Regulation of Methadone Treatment* (Washington: National Academy of Sciences Press, 1995).

20. Christopher S. Wren, "One of Medicine's Best Kept Secrets: Methadone Works," *New York Times*, June 3, 1997. D. M. Novick and J. Herman, "Medical Maintenance: The Treatment of Chronic Opiate Dependence in General Medical Practice," *Journal of Substance Abuse Treatment* 8 (1991): 233–239.

21. G. H. Dunteman, W. S. Condelli, and J. A. Fairbanks, "Predicting Cocaine Use among Methadone Patients: Analysis of Findings from a National Study," *Hospital and Community Psychiatry* 43 (1992): 608–611.

22. D. D. Simpson and H. J. Friend, "Legal Status and Long-term Outcomes for Addicts in the DARP Follow-up Project," in C. G. Leukefeld and F. M. Tims, eds., *Compulsory Treatment of Drug Abuse: Research and*

Clinical Practice, NIDA Research Monograph no. 86 (U.S. Department of Health and Human Services, 1988), 81–98.

23. D. D. Simpson and G. W. Joe, "Treatment Retention and Follow-Up Outcomes in the Drug Abuse Treatment Outcome Study (DATOS)," *Psychology of Addictive Behavior* 11, no. 4 (1997): 294–307.

24. D. D. Simpson and S. B. Sells, "Effectiveness of Treatment for Drug Abuse: An Overview of the DARP Research Program," *Advances in Alcohol and Substance Abuse* 2 (1983): 7–29.

25. G. DeLeon et al., "The Therapeutic Community: Success and Improvement Rates Five Years after Treatment," *International Journal of Addictions* 17 (1982): 703–747.

26. Denise Grady, "Engineered Mice Mimic Drug Mental Ills," *New York Times,* Feb. 20, 1996, C1.

27. Simpson and Sells, "Effectiveness of Treatment."

28. M. D. Anglin, "Efficacy of Civil Commitment in Treating Narcotics Addiction," *Journal of Drug Issues* 18 (1988): 527–545.

29. Personal communication, Paul Denia, research director of Brooklyn DTAP, Kings County District Attorney's Office. Also Charles J. Haynes, Kings County district attorney, "DTAP Seventh Annual Report" (Oct. 1996–Oct. 1997).

30. Urban Institute, "Recent Findings from the Evaluation of the D.C. Superior Court Drug Intervention Program," May 1997. Focus-group comment in personal communication, Adele Harrell, senior researcher, Urban Institute.

31. Bureau of Justice Statistics, "Recidivism of Felons on Probation, 1986–89," Special Report, U.S. Department of Justice, Office of Justice Programs, 1992.

32. General Accounting Office, U.S. Congress, "Social Security: Disability Benefits for Drug Addicts and Alcoholics Are out of Control," report no. T-HEHS-94–101 (Washington).

33. P. M. Miller, "A Behavioral Intervention Program for Chronic Public Drunkenness Offenders," *Archives of General Psychiatry* 32 (1975): 915–918.

34. S. T. Higgins et al., "Incentives Improve Outcome in Outpatient Behavioral Treatment of Cocaine Dependence," *Archives of General Psychiatry* 51 (1994): 568–576. K. Silverman et al., "Voucher-based Reinforcement of Attendance by Unemployed Methadone Patients in a Job Skills Training Program," *Drug and Alcohol Dependence* 41 (1996): 197–207.

35. Congressional Research Service Memorandum, "Prevalence of Drug Use among Welfare Recipients," June 6, 1997.

If Addiction Is Involuntary, How Can Punishment Help?

5

George E. Vaillant

Speak roughly to your little boy,
And beat him when he sneezes.
He only does it to annoy,
Because he knows it teases.

Lewis Carroll

Addiction to drugs, whether heroin, nicotine, or alcohol, has been viewed as a disease rather than an act of free will. The reason for this viewpoint is that the neural circuitry underlying much of addiction is nearly as involuntary (that is, beyond conscious control) as sneezing, or vomiting, or falling asleep while driving. Beatings, mandatory sentencing, and the firm knowledge that falling asleep on a superhighway may be fatal have little effect on such behavior because in each instance the brain is "on automatic pilot."

Put differently, the sequence of linked behaviors leading the addict back into addiction is analogous to a neural avalanche. Once the sequence of linked neural and behavioral events is fully under way, intervention is often futile. Thus, although addiction is often called a "disease," doctors are as powerless in the face of addiction as is the criminal justice system. The solution is to have a *structure* in place to abort the avalanche. If neither law (predicated on free will) nor medicine (predicated on an altered biology that can be ameliorated) alone is effective, how should society provide a structure to abort relapse? One answer is to appreciate that behavior is a function of its consequences—but of its *short-term,* not its *long-term* consequences.

A second and related answer is that society must evolve the same paternalistic controls over drug abuse that it has evolved for truancy and suicide. By this I mean that society, with suitable safeguards, must

144

defy John Stuart Mill, who maintained that coercion should not be employed for an individual's own good. Society must impose structure, but structure that is both implacably coercive *and* reinforcing. Equally important, the coercive structure must be voluntarily assented to. The rigors of law school and of marriage offer everyday examples of voluntary but coercive structures. In this chapter I will first pose the problem of relapse prevention, next offer illustrated examples of successful "coercive" interventions, and finally present the critical components of such successful structures.

Who Is Responsible for Addiction?

Before focusing on relapse prevention, why does not society just prevent addiction from beginning? Why should people behave so self-destructively as to become addicted in the first place? It is easy to shift responsibility for self-detrimental human behavior from scapegoat to scapegoat. Thus, in the realm of delinquency (and heroin abuse), society goes from one verse of *West Side Story*'s memorable song "Gee, Officer Krupke" to the next. The delinquent is lazy *or* deserving *or* bad *or* victimized. It is the same with the causes of addiction.

American society between 1910 and 1920 regarded both alcohol and drug abuse as self-indulgent sins to be eradicated; all that was needed was to legislate morality (Terry and Pellens 1970). In 1914 the Harrison Act was passed to abolish opiate abuse, and in 1919 the Volstead Act was passed to abolish alcohol abuse. These laws failed, and in the 1930s the scapegoats shifted. Addiction was not a sin; the enemy were the bootleggers and the evil Mafia pushers and the irresponsible doctors who addicted the innocent. This attribution, too, failed, so in the 1940s blame was shifted from society to the drug. It was the special pharmacological properties of heroin that were dangerous. Addiction was a disease, and detoxification was its cure. Detoxification, too, proved a failure; for as Mark Twain observed with regard to smoking, stopping (that is, detoxification) was so easy he had done it 20 times.

More recently, it has become clear that neither the Mob nor the addicting properties of drugs nor sinful human nature is the main cause of addiction in the United States. Thus it has become popular to shift responsibility for addiction onto society. If society just does its part, addiction will be solved. So on the one hand, a guilty society allocates more funds for clinics and welfare and school drug-education programs; and on the other hand, an angry society allocates more funds for high-security prisons and enforcement of the narcotics laws. But reassigning blame solves nothing. Rates of addiction continue to climb. As of the beginning of the twenty-first century we know much more about treating addiction than about preventing it.

Shifting Attention from Prevention to Treatment

If efforts to prevent addiction have failed, we can at least figure out how to treat it. In making this shift in focus, it is important to remember that the skills involved in climbing out of a hole are different from the skills that allow us not to fall into holes in the first place. If the sales of cigarettes, alcohol, and heroin have not fallen, an astonishingly large number of addicts recover every year. Why? Empirically, in combating addiction, four methods—parole (Vaillant 1988), employee assistance programs (EAPs; Walsh et al. 1991), methadone maintenance, and self-help groups (Vaillant 1995)—have enjoyed the greatest success. Why? Perhaps because they all avoid blame but employ coercion. All appreciate that behavior is a function of its short-term consequences. In that sense all four are like neither medicine nor the law. Unlike the law, they do not blame the individual for cause, and unlike medicine, they coerce the individual into responsibility for cure. All four programs work *with* the addict, not *on* him; but, paradoxically, they all support individual autonomy by infringing upon the addict's right to engage in self-detrimental behavior. They all require that the addict experience the consequences of his behavior, but in a way that permits him to change. None has much faith in free will; all have faith in submission to involuntary behavior modification. All are coercive—but only with the addict's permission.

Our prohibitions against truancy and suicide provide the most obvious examples of society's infringing on individual liberty for the "good" of the individual rather than of society. To be effective such interventions must be carried out not by conventional caregivers but by a good-hearted criminal justice system. The policeman, not the psychiatrist, crawls out on the ledge of the tall building, and the truant officer, not a social worker, comes to the playground. But their aim is to help, not punish.

We cannot hope to stamp out addiction or truancy or suicide by appeal to reason. Successful interventions in the addictions demand that we focus upon irrationalities common to all self-destructive people. Admittedly, it is a delicate balancing act. The task is to make individuals responsible for their own irrational motivation. Such *irrational motivation* goes by many different names: conditioned behavior, self-punitive expression of anger, bad genes, poor self-esteem, maladaptive ego mechanisms of defense, and undersocialization.

An example of irrational motivation is illustrated by the fact that the consumption of drugs that are used socially (that is, rationally) is highly price sensitive. Consumption of drugs that are used addictively (that is, self-destructively) is quite price insensitive (Vaillant 1995). After the Harrison Act outlawed the over-the-counter sale of narcotics in America, more than a hundred thousand middle-aged hypochondriacal but rational women gave up dependence on opiates (Terry and Pellens 1970). But the passage of the Harrison Act probably did not significantly affect the prevalence of hitherto legal heroin dependence among miserable, delinquent, unemployed young men (Lichtenstein 1914). Free education does not cure truancy; that can only be done by coercive structure.

The Carrot and the Stick

Both the conventional criminal justice model and the conventional medical model are quite unable to integrate caring and coercive strategies. Indeed, many caretakers and social workers (liberals) in our communities are at war with the stick-wielding disciplinarians and police (conservatives). Unlike a good football coach, society does not know how *simultaneously* to "reward" (put the client first) and to "kick ass" (enforce good behavior by coercive sanctions). Too often, both drunks and truants—in need of integrated care and discipline—are sent off *either* to jails or to clinics. Both fail miserably.

For example, "liberals" often insist upon a juvenile criminal addict's record being sealed when he reaches his 18th birthday. This makes it impossible for judges to make intelligent sentencing decisions until the youth has had the time to reestablish an adult criminal track record, when it is usually too late. This is as foolish as denying a doctor access to an adult diabetic's adolescent medical record. On the other hand, the "conservative" mandatory sentences (such as "three strikes and you're out") throw away the power of parole—arguably the most powerful therapeutic tool for care that criminal justice possesses (Sampson and Laub 1993).

Let me offer employee assistance programs (EAPs) as an initial model for integrating the carrot and the stick. By coercive structured behavior modification I do not mean regimens like those in *1984* or *Clockwork Orange,* I mean union-management partnerships that use the threat of job loss to coerce employees with problems to submit to clinical treatment and supervision for their own good. Fundamental to EAPs is the principle "We will protect your job but only if you behave in ways that will help to overcome your dependency on drugs." Historically, EAPs evolved out of the Occupational Alcoholism Programs that began in the 1940s, especially in the automobile industry. In the 1980s the Drug Free Work Place Act of 1988 encouraged still further expansion. At present, 90 percent of the Fortune 1000 companies have EAPs (Masi 1994). Discipline in EAPs is tough, but it is fairly administered and highly predictable. Employees' continued employment depends upon their compliance with recommended treatment regimens. But the success of such employee assistance programs defies simple logic and depends on coerced, involuntary behavior modification to which the client acquiesces.

On the one hand, discipline in a medical clinic is nonexistent. The most caring family physician or psychotherapist is quite powerless over a patient's fatal cigarette habit. On the other hand, the discipline in jails is powerful but too often unpredictable; such discipline is punitive and not short-term. Jails fail to provide the element of care and choice essential to individual reform. Psychiatric commitment laws, truancy laws, and union-blessed EAP sanctions have been decided democratically. Models for democratically determined, but coercively enforced, "smoke-free workplaces" are facilitating smoking cessation.

Let me step back a little to underscore both the importance of and the resistance to such coercion. At first glance, we consider societal interventions in truancy and suicide as uncontroversial as submitting to the coercive structure of law school, matrimony, or the Marine Corps. Before tuberculosis was brought under control, every Harvard University faculty member had to submit to a state-mandated chest X-ray every three years as a condition of employment. The carrot was that if found infected, the faculty member was granted paid sick leave. The stick was that the X-rays and treatment were mandatory if the faculty member wished to remain on the payroll. Although the rules were promulgated by the state board of health, the Harvard faculty—Christian scientists included—willingly came under the control of economic behavior modification. The ACLU did not intervene.

The question is, can we respond to narcotic addiction in the same way that we do to truancy and suicide without seriously violating the individual's civil liberties? Certainly, legislative answers to difficult social problems evolve; they rarely emerge by fiat. Before a delicate balance between law, medicine, and self-determination was arrived at, melancholics were burned as witches by the clergy, hanged as attempted self-murderers by the judges, and bled to death by high-minded physicians.

The Integration of Care and Coercion

Suppose that we cease to conceptualize drug addiction as reflecting disease *or* societal discrimination *or* moral turpitude. Suppose that we conceive of drug addiction as a whole constellation of conditioned but unconscious behaviors. Then the relative success of coercion over conventional psychiatric intervention begins to make sense. Like the melancholic rescued by police from a building ledge, addicts, once order is restored to their lives, become less self-destructive. Addicts, whether they are victims of prejudice and multiproblem families or whether they are overprivileged physicians, need structure, not insight and willpower, if they are to change their addictive behavior. Let me illustrate this bold generalization with a few examples.

These three illustrative structures were all provided by "voluntary" but highly coercive means: the army, parole, and methadone maintenance. The examples are all drawn from a prospective study of the natural history of New York City heroin addicts. All support the argument that, in effecting recovery, structure (the carrot *and* the stick) is more powerful than either coercion or care alone.

Example 1: Compulsory Employment

The first example illustrates the effect of military service. Figure 5.1 is a composite graph of the employment careers of 50 New York City heroin abusers (Vaillant 1966a). They were of above-average intelligence and were admitted to the U.S. Public Health Service in Lexington, Kentucky, in 1952; 54 percent were African American. Largely derived from their social security records, the figure shows the proportion of these 50 addicts who were employed at any given age. Military duty was ascertained from other sources.

These 50 addicts were selected for special study because they were born between 1920 and 1924—the critical birth cohort to examine the special structure that existed for young men during World War II.

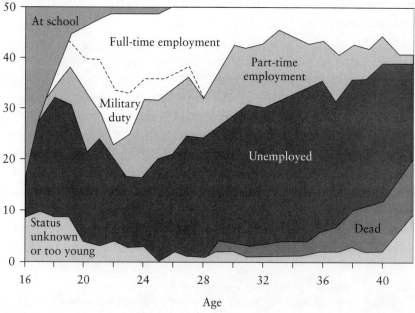

Figure 5.1. Employment careers of 50 New York City heroin abusers admitted to the U.S. Public Health Service in Lexington, Kentucky, in 1952: proportion employed, by age. Source: Vaillant 1966a.

First, restrictions on world trade meant that from 1940 to 1945 heroin importation into New York City was almost impossible. Thus only five of these men became addicted to heroin prior to the end of World War II. Second, a booming war economy and universal military service led to full employment—even for disadvantaged minority groups. Nevertheless, even during the special conditions of World War II, over half of these future heroin addicts were jobless or working part-time. In short, their inability to work was not a result of heroin addiction, nor of the economy, nor of bias. Even before addiction, these intelligent, able-bodied men without major mental illness had difficulty remaining employed. Put differently, the figure supports the medical model: these men's inability to work had more to do with individual deficits (such as situational depression, personality disorder, or undersocialization by dysfunctional families) than with societal deficits (such as addiction or bigotry or economic conditions).

However, the figure also illustrates the power of coercion. Prior to age 40, these men spent a significant proportion of their employed time within the structured coercive setting of the military. If you have been very deprived as a child, army life offers as many carrots as it does sticks. Other men, unable to find work even during the favorable conditions of World War II, found regular employment after age 40 but only when work was made a condition of their parole from state penitentiaries. For these men, employment was again due to their acceptance of coercion.

Coercion, however, works only when it has meaning to the individual. Making heroin illegal seems quite meaningless to depressed undersocialized adolescents, for opiates can compete with the best antidepressants on the market. In contrast, compelling people to join the army during a just war or insisting upon work in order to maintain parole from a state penitentiary has meaning. Similarly, society can pass enforceable laws against suicide and truancy, because they seem meaningful.

Example 2: Parole
The importance of parole is drawn from the therapeutic vicissitudes of 100 consecutively admitted inner-city New York heroin addicts over an 18-year period (Vaillant 1966a, 1988). (Most of these men were

too young to have been included in the figure illustrating employment of older addicts during World War II.) Fifty of these addicts were white; 50 were African American. Among the two groups 30 percent were Hispanic. In 1952, at the time of their first admission to the U.S. Public Health Service Hospital in Lexington, Kentucky, 82 percent had been addicted to heroin for at least 12 months and 75 of these 100 men had been motivated to seek treatment voluntarily. The other 25 had gone to Lexington under the coercion of New York City courts. Within a year after discharge from the hospital, almost all the addicts had relapsed to the chronic use of heroin. Willpower and sympathetic medical treatment were not enough.

However, in 1964, 12 years later, 49 of these addicts were abstinent from drugs and living in the community; 30 of these addicts had achieved stable abstinences that averaged almost eight years in duration. Half were regularly employed. In 1972, twenty years after admission, only one-third of the surviving men were still addicted. What sticks and what carrots led to this eventual high rate of "cure"?

In the decade 1950–1960, both New York City and the federal government offered several facilities for voluntary, confidential withdrawal from drugs in medical settings. The 100 addicts in Table 5.1 had been particularly fortunate. First, they were all admitted to the USPHS Hospital at Lexington, which offered five months of free hospitalization and a modest amount of free psychiatric treatment, especially to motivated patients. In addition, for three years after discharge from that hospital, a social service agency tried to contact them at regular intervals. Nevertheless, at the end of 12 years 97 of the 100 addicts had relapsed. As a group they had been voluntarily withdrawn from drugs in a medical or psychiatric setting 270 times, only to relapse 97 percent of the time. The "carrot" of humane, voluntary treatment of drug addiction had proven worthless.

Also during the decade 1950–1960, state and federal law enforcement agencies were responding to a wave of concern generated by the publicized postwar rise in narcotic addiction among urban youth. The sale or possession of narcotics met with stiff penalties. Between 1952 and 1964 the 100 "underclass" addicts in this study were also treated harshly as criminals. They were sent to jail for one to eight months on a total of 279 occasions. Again, 97 percent of these jail sentences

Table 5.1 Relative efficacy of five modes of "treatment" in facilitating abstinences of a year or more: 100 heroin addicts

	1952–1964		1965–1970	
	"Treatment" exposures*	% followed by abstinence	"Treatment" exposures*	% followed by abstinence
Voluntary hospitali- zation	270	3	91	2
Short im- prisonment (<9 mo)	279	3	84	3
Long im- prisonment (>9 mo)	46	13	4	25
Prison and parole	30	67	4	100
Methadone mainten- ance			15	67

Source: Vaillant 1988.
*Over 18 years 90% of the 100 addicts encountered several of the listed types of treatment.

failed to deter relapse to addiction even for a year. In other words, only 3 percent of short imprisonments or short hospitalizations were followed by abstinence from narcotics for a year or more. On 50 occasions during the 18-year follow-up period the 100 addicts were imprisoned for nine months to three years without significant parole. Even with such prolonged institutionalization, 87 percent still relapsed within a year. In short, the "stick" of criminal justice had proved equally worthless.

The treatment of alcohol abuse is no different. Voluntary methods and willpower are little help. Legalizing alcohol (a solution often advocated to control heroin addiction) by repealing the Volstead Act in 1932 doubled both the number of alcoholics and their death rate from cirrhosis (Vaillant 1995). During the 1980s, providing alcoholics with a "carrot" of insurance that paid for hospitalizations of 14–28 days did little to alter the natural course of alcoholic dependence (Vaillant 1995). For there was no "stick" to help prevent relapse when the hospitalized alcoholics returned to the community. Nor does it help just to punish alcohol abuse. Mandating Antabuse (disulfiram: a drug that causes even one drink to result in severe physical discomfort) becomes ineffective after a year (Mottin 1973). For like mandated prison sentences for heroin abuse, Antabuse, like the "stick" alone, offers the alcoholic no "carrot" to replace the alcohol that has been taken away.

Fortunately for the 100 addicts in Table 5.1, there were two other kinds of treatment experiences—parole and methadone maintenance. Both were coercive and both were caring. Both took away what was self-destructive, and both offered a caring substitute in return. No addict who failed with either of these treatments succeeded after short hospitalization or short imprisonment alone.

During the 18-year period of follow-up 26 of the 100 addicts had received at least nine months of imprisonment followed by at least a year of parole; 8 of the 26 had had two such experiences, for a total of 34 instances of prison and parole. By definition such severe sentences were given to the most "undeserving" and antisocial addicts. But in-the-community abstinences of a year or more resulted from 24 such experiences, and in at least 11 cases, once parole was terminated the addicts continued to maintain employment. But this therapeutic effect of parole was quite unintentional.

Each man could serve as his own control. Prior to receiving parole, all 34 of these men had received other forms of treatment, and all had relapsed. Eighty percent had relapsed after hospitalization and 55 percent after short imprisonment. They received parole, however, only because of the length of their sentences. The law had intended only to punish these men severely—either for repeated felonies or for large sales of narcotics. The men's recovery from addiction during parole was unexpected.

But successful parole did not demand that the addict abandon one habit without providing him with an alternative habit. Parole provided a fairly rigidly defined schedule of competing behaviors to the one the addict had formerly pursued. To keep his parole the addict not only had to avoid certain of his associates but also had to maintain both stable employment and contact with a helpful, powerful authority figure. Each week he had to show his pay stub to his parole officer. Even among addicts with the poorest previous work histories, the correlation between parole and employment was dramatic. The foes of social Calvinism may overlook the fact that work can reflect competence, social utility, and self-esteem. Prior work history is one of the most powerful predictors of recovery from drug addiction (Vaillant 1966c), from delinquency (Glueck and Glueck 1943), and from alcoholism (Costello 1975). Sampson and Laub (1993) have also shown in their groundbreaking book *Crime in the Making* the power of reestablishing social bonds, of which a stable job is a prime component, to heal extremely socially alienated adolescents.

As Sampson and Laub note, the therapeutic element of the prison-parole combination appeared to rest with the parole, not the institutionalization. Prolonged compulsory supervision in the community reforms; mandatory jail sentences do not. Nevertheless, the structure of community supervision must have teeth. Truancy laws are only as good as the perseverance of the truant officer.

Ten other addicts from the study whose remission is not reflected in Table 5.1 remained abstinent for a year or more following compulsory supervision without long imprisonment. Five were under conventional court probation, one under the supervision of his county medical society, and two under the supervision of fundamentalist religious groups, and the last two were abstinent while in the army.

In interpreting the success of the compulsory supervision of addicts, it is important to bear six points in mind. First, in terms of their clinical and criminal histories, the 26 addicts in Table 5.1 who received parole were not a prognostically more favorable group. By this I mean they were not better educated, less criminal or addicted, or blessed with better premorbid work histories than addicts who did not receive parole. Table 5.2 contrasts addicts with and without parole for the seven premorbid variables most associated with good outcome. Using the chi-square test with Yates correction, there were no statistically significant differences between the two groups for any of the variables (Vaillant 1966c).

Second, age may have been one factor that enhanced the success of parole. By the time that these addicts received sentences of sufficient severity to merit parole, they were about 30 years old. Evidence from

Table 5.2   Comparison of premorbid variables for heroin addicts with and without parole

Factors	Addicts with parole n = 26	Addicts without parole n = 74
Graduated from high school	12%	22%
Served in the military	54%	43%
4+ years of employment prior to hospitalization	23%	19%
No opiates before age 21	46%	38%
First addicted <3 years before hospitalization	73%	57%
No permanent loss of a parent before age 6	77%	70%
No parent-child cultural disparity*	42%	36%

*Cultural disparity means that an addict's parents grew up in a foreign country or in the rural South and the addict grew up in New York City.

a number of sources (Alksne, Trussel, and Elinson 1959; Diskind and Klonsky 1964; McGlothin, Anglin, and Wilson 1977) indicates that parole is less effective before age 25.

Third, and very important, after the "crutch" of parole was removed, the abstinent addicts did *not* relapse more rapidly than did other addicts who achieved a year of abstinence voluntarily. In other words, for abstinence to be maintained the abstinence does not have to be voluntary; nor does the parole have to be maintained indefinitely.

Fourth, the coercion (whether via the army or via parole) was chosen by the addict; this is in contrast to some civil commitment programs. The distinction is subtle but important. This element of choice, of course, is also integral to the success of employee assistance programs. If your employer or your police chief says that you must be supervised because you use drugs, this may seem unreasonable. If your employer says you have to be supervised because of poor work performance, or the judge trades you the rigors of parole for a shortened jail time for a bank robbery, the coercion may seem reasonable.

Fifth, the biggest difference between parole officers and social workers is not that the former seem to care less, but that they have the power to care more. Society sometimes forgets that acutely suicidal patients must usually be taken to hospitals against their will by police officers, not by nurses or doctors who are untrained in coercion.

Sixth, another reason parole is more effective than psychiatric intervention is that "treatment" in the medical model can never occupy more than a few hours of an addict's week. In contrast, a parole-mandated job lasts 40 hours. (Under the incentive of parole, ex-addicts-felons living in inner-city neighborhoods with high rates of unemployment did not seem to encounter insuperable difficulty in finding and maintaining regular employment.)

Admittedly, the 1950s and early 1960s were different from today. In the 1950s, many of the addicts were shooting very expensive diluted heroin. Today, the street prices of very pure heroin are relatively low. In addition, urban unemployment and violent crime rates are higher today; most parolees are returning to more disordered neighborhoods; and the criminal justice system is more overextended. By all accounts, the quality and intensity of parole supervision in the community have declined. But that does not mean the situation has to stay that way.

The Pros and Cons of Civil Commitment

In the United States there have been two major efforts to evaluate the effects of coercion in reducing drug abuse and facilitating subsequent employment: the 1961 California Civil Addict Program or CAP (Mc-Glothin, Anglin, and Wilson 1977; Anglin 1988; Kramer and Bass 1969) and the 1966 New York Narcotic Control Commission or NACC (Inciardi 1986). These programs and similar less comprehensive efforts are reviewed in more detail elsewhere (Leukefeld and Tims 1988). Similar programs have been instituted with much greater success for physician addicts (Jones 1958; Talbott 1995).

Initiated in 1960 by the state of California, CAP provided involuntary commitment for narcotic addicts (without other criminal charges) followed by prolonged parole for both civil and criminal commitments. Inpatient treatment was conducted in a center at Corona, run by the California Department of Corrections. The guards were armed, and to escape past the barbed-wire fences was a felony. After release from the institutional phase, which was rather inflexible, the addict had to undergo a period of compulsory supervision—from one to seven years, depending on his commitment. This supervision was by a parole officer with a caseload of approximately 33 individuals. During the period of supervision the addict was expected to work regularly and to undergo frequent urine testing for illicit drug use. If the addict violated the terms of the parole, he could, on the recommendation of his parole board, be reinstitutionalized. After three years of successful community adjustment, addicts were released from their commitment.

In contrast to other civil commitment programs, the CAP program enjoyed a low caseload per parole officer, compulsory urine testing, and the capacity for rapid response if an individual returned to narcotics. However, employment was neither mandatory nor assessed. During two years of community life the 289 men with civil commitment used narcotics 22 percent of the time (Gerstein 1992). In contrast, during two years of follow-up the 292 matched controls used narcotics 50 percent of the time. Ten years later, the treatment group—three years after termination of supervision—used narcotics 17 percent of the time, while the controls used narcotics 27 percent of the time. Close community supervision and rigorous urine testing appeared to be the most important factors leading to the differences in outcome (Anglin 1988). Although 13 months of institutionalization is a steep human price to pay for such results, the Corona results were still 10 times better than those obtained by imprisonment or therapy alone (Alksne, Trussel, and Elinson 1959; Duvall, Locke, and Brill 1963).

A contrasting and less successful program of coercion was the New York Narcotic Control Commission (NACC). The NACC, which offered compulsory supervision to over 4,000 addicts and cost over $300 million, was a failure. Indeed, the ill-fated effort serves as a model of how not to conduct compulsory supervision. The NACC caseworkers had much higher caseloads than those in the California program. In addition, they lacked the power to arrest; and they did not employ urine testing to determine relapse. Thus the abscondence rates for the NACC clients were 12 times higher than for men on parole for criminal offenses.

There are several possible explanations why these deliberate programs seemed less successful than the serendipitous results noted in

Table 5.1. First, men who absconded from the CAP and NACC programs for reasons other than relapse, or who after a second admission succeeded, were still scored as relapses. In contrast, in my 20-year follow-up, I noted all the eventual successes. Second, the addicts in my study who received parole were considerably older than the average addicts in the civil commitment programs. Third, for the Lexington addicts the parole for their *criminal* offenses was more effectively enforced than the supervision provided by *civil* commitment programs for the CAP and NACC addicts. Finally, there may have been adverse selection of the clients in CAP. Both doctors and judges confuse the dimension *voluntary-involuntary* with the dimension *therapeutic-punitive*. Thus undoubtedly California doctors were reluctant to commit addicts with good prognosis to the CAP program because they could not believe coercion could be caring (Gerstein 1992).

Example 3: Methadone Maintenance

During the years 1964–1970 New York saw the introduction of methadone maintenance programs. After 1964, 15 of the 40 still chronically addicted men in Table 5.1 received methadone maintenance. Thus it was possible to study the effects of this newer treatment on a sample of 100 addicts already exposed for 12 years to a variety of other interventions. Ten of the 15 addicts who received methadone maintenance achieved stable social adjustment and freedom from illicit drug use for at least 18 months and for an average of 3 years; 5 of these men were also working. All 10 of the methadone successes had failed to become abstinent from heroin after *both* imprisonment and voluntary hospitalization. Indeed, the average previous treatment experience for each methadone success was one long imprisonment, five short imprisonments, and nine voluntary hospitalizations—all followed by relapse within a year. None of the five methadone failures had ever responded to any form of treatment, including five exposures to parole. Arguably, methadone maintenance programs are the most effective method society currently has for inducing abstinence from heroin in unselected populations (Dole, Nyswander, and Warner 1968).

At first glance, methadone maintenance would appear an example of just a "carrot." Analogous to the compulsory employment of parole, methadone maintenance takes advantage of the fact that the best way to stop a bad habit is not to forbid it out of hand but to provide a less noxious, but still gratifying, substitute. To many it was counterintuitive that helping the addict remain addicted would be helpful. Yet methadone, like parole and the military, also provides a "stick." The very fact that the addict is addicted to methadone coerces the addict to remain closely tied to a treatment facility.

How Can the Criminal Justice System Integrate Care and Coercion?

Evidence from the three examples suggests that addicts will experience the best chance of recovery when the following four conditions are met:

- When they remain in a community setting where they receive *compulsory supervision* to deter relapse and to maintain structure and employment. If such structured programs demand regular compulsory employment, they do so in a setting of the individual's choosing.
- When they are permitted some *substitute dependencies*—preferably dependence on humans rather than chemicals.
- Where new, non-guilt-provoking, sustaining *intimate relationships* are provided (for example, therapeutic communities, 12-Stepping, remarriage).
- When coercion is compatible with the addict's own value system. Usually this is accomplished through *inspirational self-help groups* rather than methadone or parole (Duvall, Locke, and Brill 1963).

Table 5.3 illustrates the importance of these four general conditions in the prevention of relapse. The left-hand column of the table shows the determinants of abstinence of a year or more in a naturalistic study of alcohol abusers who were not patients. These men were identified in a study of 400 schoolboys who were followed from age 14 to 47 (Vaillant 1995; Glueck and Glueck 1943, 1950). At some point 110 men developed alcohol abuse. Of those 110 alcohol abusers, 49 became abstinent for a year or more. In only 30 percent of the cases

Table 5.3   Conditions associated with absence of relapse for a year or more

	Untreated abstinent alcoholics (n = 49)	Treated abstinent heroin addicts (n = 30)	Treated abstinent alcoholics (n = 29)
Compulsory supervision	49%	47%	34%
Substitute dependencies	53%	60%	55%
Sustaining intimate relationships	32%	63%	31%
Inspirational self-help groups	49%	~20%*	62%

*During the period of follow-up (1952–1970) Narcotics Anonymous and self-help groups were not yet well established. Three addicts, however, became involved in fundamentalist religion or self-help groups, and three became employed in agencies helping other addicts.

was this year of abstinence associated with any sort of alcohol clinic attendance or hospitalization. But most of them experienced at least two of the conditions in Table 5.3.

The middle column shows the importance of the four conditions to sustain abstinence in the heroin addicts already discussed. The right-hand column shows the importance of the four conditions in sustained abstinence in a cohort of treated alcoholics. Recovery from addiction is anything but spontaneous. Let me examine these four general conditions in greater detail.

Compulsory Supervision

If abstinence is to be sustained, it must be maintained for years in settings closely resembling those where drugs were consumed in the past. One reason supervised abstinence (whether under parole, methadone, disulfiram, or AA) may be more enduring than voluntary abstinence achieved after hospitalization or during geographic "cures" is that supervised community abstinence occurs in the presence of many secondary reinforcers (other addicts, drug sellers, community stresses, and so on). When secondary reinforcers continue to exist, but in the absence of any reinforcement, they gradually lose their effectiveness in controlling the addict's behavior. In other words, the cascade of conditioned cues leading to relapse is replaced by an alternative cascade of cues extinguishing drugs-seeking behavior.

As we have seen, external interventions that restructure the patient's life in the community (parole, methadone maintenance, Alcoholics Anonymous) were often associated with sustained abstinence. The analogy between the treatment of addiction and that of diabetes is helpful. A diabetic's control over his illness must take place in the community through sustained self-medication with insulin, altered life habits, and conscious awareness that relapse is always possible. Such conscious awareness of the possibility of relapse is maintained by compulsory daily rituals like urine testing and diet control.

Compulsory supervision is not successful if it just punishes, but only when it alters an addict's schedule of reinforcement and provides alternative sources of gratification. For example, parole required weekly proof of employment from heroin addicts previously convinced that they could not or would not hold a job. Parole can also alter old social networks—a common source of unconscious conditioned relapse. Similarly, abstinence from alcohol is reinforced by external events that systematically and negatively alter the consequences of alcohol consumption. These events, not willpower or pious warnings about liver disease (which is painless), remind the alcoholic that alcohol is an "enemy." Such contingent events can be medical consequences (such as painful stomach problems exacerbated by alcohol consumption), or legal consequences (such as probation), or disulfiram.

Substitute Dependencies

Principles of behavior modification also help to explain why substitute dependencies (that is, competing behaviors) are useful in preventing relapse. For example, in facilitating long-term abstinence in alcohol abuse disulfiram (Antabuse) is no more effective than placebo. The reason is that disulfiram takes alcohol away but does not replace drinking with a competing behavior. In contrast, in order to keep his parole, an addicted felon must not only avoid certain of his associates but also must maintain both stable employment and contact with a helpful authority figure. Substitute dependencies can take many different forms, ranging from the somewhat maladaptive (such as chain smoking or compulsive gambling) to the clinically designed models (such as continuously sipping a glass of soda water at cocktail parties or becoming "addicted" to a methadone maintenance clinic).

Sustaining Intimate Relationships

The formation of new stable social relationships is often associated with remission in substance-abuse patients (Vaillant 1988). The most familiar example is epitomized by the barroom refrain "Wedding bells are breaking up that old gang of mine." New social networks help extinguish many of the secondary reinforcers associated with relapse. Drug-free communities like Phoenix Houses offer perhaps the best example of such networks. Such communities do not ask addicts to bond with family members toward whom, once they are abstinent, they must feel guilty, or with nonaddicts, with whom they cannot identify. Phoenix House asks the addict to bond with a group of companions whom they have not hurt, with whom they can identify, and who do not use drugs.

Inspirational Self-Help Groups

In the United States one group of coercive programs for addiction has focused exclusively on the person and virtually ignored the drug. These programs involve ex-addicts helping current addicts to abstain in a quasi-religious communal environment. Such programs were developed too late to have been important to the men depicted in Table 5.1. Phoenix House and Narcotics Anonymous are the best known examples. Review of the results from these programs reveals that they have been roughly as successful as either prolonged compulsory supervision or most methadone maintenance programs (Gerstein 1992). But, like methadone maintenance and unlike AA, these "voluntary" programs depend for their success upon a backdrop of laws forbidding the use of narcotics. Addicts often seek admission to self-help programs under direct coercion from the courts.

However, self-help programs resemble the Marine Corps more than they do either parole or methadone maintenance. Acceptance into a therapeutic community is offered as a privilege—neither as a right nor as a retribution. Like the Marine Corps, such communities ask individuals to respect a power greater than themselves. Neither sympathy nor moral judgment is provided. To remain in the program requires a 24-hour-a-day commitment and involvement. The addict is continuously confronted by his obligations to the tangible ex-addict community in which he lives. No job is too menial. But the people who invite him to scrub floors have credibility: unlike doctors and policemen, they are ex-addicts who once scrubbed those floors themselves. It is for a reason that the motto in Alcoholics Anonymous is "Identify, Don't Compare" and Marine drill instructors were once privates themselves.

Nor do self-help groups demand that the addict give up drugs without obtaining something in return. The very close-knit, quasi-familial, quasi-religious community offers in real coinage what the addict had been previously seeking in pharmacological counterfeit. In this feeling of solidarity, the Marine Corps, the Hell's Angels, and Phoenix House bear a certain resemblance to each other. Group membership also provides a "new nonstigmatized identity" that is important to sustained abstinence (Stall and Biernacki 1986). Enhanced hope and self-esteem assist addicts in maintaining abstinence.

Alcoholics Anonymous and inspirational residential communities provide the other three conditions found in naturalistic studies of relapse prevention: compulsory supervision, substitute dependencies, and sustained intimate relationships. AA provides a busy schedule of social and service activities with supportive former drinkers, especially at times of high risk (such as holidays). A requirement of AA is that a member "work the program," and as with compulsory supervision, AA encourages its members to return again and again both to group meetings and to their "sponsors."

Increasingly, compulsory supervision, substitute dependencies, sustained relationships, and inspirational self-help groups are becoming the bases of clinical relapse-prevention programs. Court-mandated commitment to therapeutic communities also effects relapse prevention through compulsory supervision, substitute dependency, self-esteem building through inspiration of group members, and drug-free social networks. Cognitive/behavioral programs (Marlatt and Gordon 1985) also provide positive feedback for facilitating the recall of alcohol-related negative experiences, finding substitutes for drinking, and developing social supports that help reinforce sobriety.

Conclusion

We must cease to conceptualize drug addiction as either just a disease or just the voluntary use of a drug to provide emotional solace or just exquisite self-indulgence. If, instead, we conceive of drug addiction as a whole constellation of conditioned, unconscious behaviors, then the relative success of parole, methadone maintenance, and Alcoholics Anonymous over conventional clinical interventions begins to make sense. These community interventions serve to impose a structure on the addict's life. This structure interferes with drug-seeking behavior based upon conditioned withdrawal symptoms and upon conditioned reinforcers like the ritual of "belting up," the friendship of hard-drinking friends, and the experience of purposeful behavior that precedes self-medication.

I am also suggesting that John Stuart Mill was too restrictive when he wrote, "The only purpose for which power can rightly be exercised over any member of a civilized community, against his will, is to prevent harm to others." I am suggesting that power may be used to prevent unintentional self-destructive behavior (drug abuse and truancy). Previous legislative policies toward suicide and truancy, and current employee assistance program policies toward alcoholism in the workplace and toward drug use by professional athletes, offer us possible models with which to move forward.

References

This work was supported by research grants KO5-MH00364, AA-01372, and MH42248 from the National Institute of Mental Health, United States Public Health Service.

Alksne, Harold, Ray E. Trussel, and Jack Elinson. 1959. "A Follow-Up Study of Treated Adolescent Narcotic Users." Report for Columbia University School of Public Health and Administrative Medicine.

Anglin, M. Douglas. 1988. "Efficacy of Civil Commitment in Treating Narcotics Addiction." *Journal of Drug Issues* 18: 527–545.

Carroll, Lewis. 1993. *Through the Looking Glass and What Alice Found There.* New York: William Morrow.

Costello, Raymond M. 1975. "Alcoholism Treatment and Evaluation: In Search of Methods." *International Journal of the Addictions* 10: 251–275.

Diskind, Meyer H., and George Klonsky. 1964. "A Second Look at the New York State Parole Drug Experiment." *Federal Probation* 28: 34.

Dole, Vincent P., Marie E. Nyswander, and Alan Warner. 1968. "Successful Treatment of 750 Criminal Addicts." *Journal of the American Medical Association* 206: 2710–11.

Duvall, Henrietta J., Benjamin Z. Locke, and Leon Brill. 1963. "Follow-Up Study of Narcotic Drug Addicts Five Years after Hospitalization." *Public Health Report* 78: 185–193.

Gerstein, Dean R. 1992. "The Effectiveness of Drug Treatment." In Charles P. O'Brien and Jerome H. Jaffe, eds., *Addictive States*. New York: Rowen Press.

Glueck, Sheldon, and Eleanor Glueck. 1943. *Criminal Careers in Retrospect.* New York: Commonwealth Fund.

———. 1950. *Unraveling Juvenile Delinquency.* New York: Commonwealth Fund.

Inciardi, James A. 1986. *The War on Drugs: Heroin, Cocaine, Crime and Public Policy.* Palo Alto: Mayfield.

Jones, Louis E. 1958. "How 92% Beat the Dope Habit." *Bulletin of the Los Angeles County Medical Association* 88, no. 7: 19, 37–40.

Kramer, John C., and Richard A. Bass. 1969. "Institutionalization Patterns among Civilly Committed Addicts." *Journal of the American Medical Association* 208: 2297–2301.

Leukefeld, Carl G., and Frank M. Tims, eds. 1988. *Compulsory Treatment of Drug Abuse: Research and Clinical Practice.* NIDA Research Monograph 86. Washington: Government Printing Office.

Lichtenstein, Perry M. 1914. "Narcotic Addiction." *New York Medical Journal* 100: 962–966.

Marlatt, G. Alan, and Judith Gordon, eds. 1985. *Relapse Prevention: Maintenance Strategies in the Treatment of Addictive Behaviors.* New York: Guilford.

Masi, Dale A. 1994. *Evaluating Your Employee Assistance and Managed Behavioral Care Program.* Troy, Mich.: Performance Resource Press.

McGlothin, William H., M. Douglas Anglin, and Bruce D. Wilson. 1977. "A Follow-Up of Admissions to the California Civil Addict Program." *American Journal of Drug and Alcohol Abuse* 4: 179–199.

Mottin, J. L. 1973. "Drug-Induced Attenuation of Alcohol Consumption." *Quarterly Journal of Studies on Alcohol* 34: 444–472.

Sampson, Robert J., and John H. Laub. 1993. *Crime in the Making.* Cambridge, Mass.: Harvard University Press.

Stall, Robb, and Patrick Biernacki. 1986. "Spontaneous Remission from the Problematic Use of Substances: An Inductive Model Derived from a Comparative Analysis of the Alcohol, Opiate, Tobacco and Food/Obesity Literatures." *International Journal of the Addictions* 21: 1–23.

Talbott, G. Douglas. 1995. "Reducing Relapse in Health Providers and Professionals." *Psychiatric Annals* 25: 669–672.

Terry, Charles E., and Mildred Pellens. 1970. *The Opium Problem.* Montclair, N.J.: Paterson Smith.

Vaillant, George E. 1966a. "A 12-Year Follow-Up of New York Narcotic Addicts: I. The Relation of Treatment to Outcome." *American Journal of Psychiatry* 122: 727–737.

———. 1966b. "A 12-Year Follow-up of New York Narcotic Addicts: II. The Natural History of a Chronic Disease." *New England Journal of Medicine* 275: 1282–88.

———. 1966c. "A 12-Year Follow-up of New York Narcotic Addicts: IV. Some Characteristics and Determinants of Abstinence." *American Journal of Psychiatry* 123: 573–584.

———. 1988. "What Can Long-Term Follow-Up Teach Us about Relapse and Prevention of Relapse in Addiction?" *British Journal of Addiction* 83: 1147–57.

———. 1995. *The Natural History of Alcoholism, Revisited.* Cambridge, Mass.: Harvard University Press.

Walsh, Diana C., et al. 1991. "A Randomized Trial of Treatment Options for Alcohol-Abusing Workers." *New England Journal of Medicine* 325: 775–782.

Controlling Drug Use and Crime
with Testing, Sanctions, and Treatment

6

Mark A. R. Kleiman

Crime—at least crime of the sort which often leads to arrest and punishment—tends to attract those who are reckless and impulsive, rather than those who fit the model of self-interested rationality. That simple observation has strong implications for efforts aimed at both deterrence and rehabilitation, but those implications have either not been drawn or not been acted on. Moreover, the obvious opposition of interest between offenders and everyone else has been allowed to conceal from the public consciousness the common interest in improving offenders' capacities for self-command.

The relatively small number of offenders who are frequent, high-dose users of cocaine, heroin, and methamphetamine (no more than 3 million all told)[1] account for such a large proportion both of crime and of the money spent on illicit drugs that getting a handle on their behavior is inseparable from getting a handle on street crime and the drug markets. Yet current policies for dealing with them ignore everything we know both about addiction and about deterrence. For the reckless and impulsive, deferred and low-probability threats of severe punishment are less effective than immediate and high-probability threats of mild punishment. By contrast, current practices for dealing with offenders over-rely on severity at the sacrifice of certainty and immediacy.

The probation and parole systems are the key to managing the population of drug-using offenders. Abstinence from drug use ought to be made a condition of continued liberty, and that condition ought to be enforced with frequent drug tests and predictable sanctions, with treatment required or offered to those whose repeated failure to abstain under coercion alone shows them to be in need of it.

The benefits of mounting such a program would vastly outstrip its costs, and outstrip the benefits of any other program that could be mounted against drugs and crime using comparable resources. The administrative and political barriers are formidable but perhaps not insurmountable.

Background

The damage associated with illicit drugs is impressive:

- several million dependent users[2]
- an illicit industry generating tens of billions of dollars in revenue[3]
- recent cocaine or heroin use by nearly half of all those arrested for serious crimes in big cities[4]
- hundreds of thousands of people, many of them very young, regularly committing felony drug-selling offenses[5]
- enormous amounts of violence associated with drug transactions, or at least with weapons obtained for use in, and with the proceeds of, drug selling;
- neighborhood disruption due to the disorder and violence of open illicit markets;
- $25 billion spent on drug law enforcement, out of a total national enforcement budget of $125 billion;[6]
- 350,000 persons behind bars for drug sales or possession[7] out of a total national prison-plus-jail population of 1.65 million;[8]
- injection drug use a strong second to sex in the transmission of HIV.[9]

All of this damage is highly concentrated in poor, urban neighborhoods with primarily ethnic-minority populations. (Two-thirds of those admitted to state prisons for drug offenses are African American.)[10]

Offenders make an enormous financial contribution to the illicit drug-dealing industries, with all their undesirable side effects: violence, disorder, corruption, enforcement expense, imprisonment, and the diversion of adolescents in poor urban neighborhoods away from school and licit work and toward drug dealing. The numbers are rather startling.

About four-fifths of the cocaine and heroin sold is consumed by heavy, rather than casual, users. (The precise proportion depends on the definition of the term "heavy," but all of the plausible definitions have to do with people who spend more than $10,000 per year on their chosen drugs; for cocaine, this group accounts for somewhere between one-fifth and one-quarter of all the past-month users.[11]) This highly skewed distribution of consumption accords with the general heuristic principle known as Pareto's Law (which holds that 80 percent of the volume of any activity is accounted for by 20 percent of the participants) and with what is known about the distribution of alcohol consumption.[12] It is also supported by a comparison of consumption-based and enforcement-based estimates of cocaine volumes: a projection of cocaine users' reports on how much they consume from the National Household Survey on Drug Abuse accounts for only about 30 metric tons of cocaine a year, while enforcement data suggest total consumption of about 300 metric tons.[13]

That gap implies the existence of an unmeasured hard core which uses the bulk of the cocaine. No plausible definition of "casual" use, multiplied by the survey-estimated number of users, could account for any substantial proportion of the $30 billion estimated annual cocaine market.[14]

Statistics from the Arrestee Drug Abuse Monitoring (ADAM) system suggest that the "hidden" population of heavy users consists largely of frequent offenders.[15] While not all of those who are arrested and who test positive for cocaine are heavy users, the short "detection window" for the urine monitoring of cocaine use (48–72 hours) means that heavy users are likely to account for most of the positive post-arrest tests. By one calculation, about 1.7 million different heavy cocaine users are arrested for felonies in any given year, or about three-quarters of the estimated 2.2 million total heavy users.[16] When not in prison or jail, these user/offenders tend to be on probation or parole.

If heavy users account for 80 percent of the cocaine, and if three-quarters of them are in the criminal justice population, then 60 percent of the total cocaine is sold to persons under (nominal) criminal justice supervision. Therefore any short-to-medium-term effort aimed at reducing demand for cocaine must focus on this group, on the principle that if you're going duck hunting you have to go where the ducks are.

Conversely, though most users of illicit drugs are not otherwise lawbreakers, continued use of expensive drugs by those who pay for their habits from the proceeds of their crimes virtually guarantees continued criminal activity. Among offenders, the use of expensive drugs predicts both high-rate offending and persistence in crime. Therefore any policy to deal with high-rate offenders needs to address their substance abuse problems. Thus, whether our concern is crime generally or the abuse of illicit drugs, we are drawn to consider policies for dealing with the behavior of a relatively small number of high-volume user/offenders.

Current Policies

Neither current drug policies nor current correctional policies offer any real hope of substantially reducing drug consumption by user/offenders. The drug-policy triad of prevention-enforcement-treatment is largely irrelevant. Let's take its elements in order.

First, prevention. Not only is it obviously futile to prevent what has already occurred, there is no evidence that the standard array of either school-based or media-based drug-prevention messages have much to say to those who are likely to develop into drug-involved offenders in the future, as opposed to the middle-class kids whose parents' concerns dominate the politics of drug policy and especially the politics of the prevention effort.[17] (A focus on preventing drug *dealing*, using some mix of messages to change attitudes and other policies to shrink dealing opportunities, might be more relevant, but that idea is nowhere near the policy agenda.)[18]

Second, enforcement. By making drugs more expensive and harder to obtain, enforcement can reduce both consumption by current users and the initiation rate. Compared with the hypothetical baselines of either legalization or zero enforcement, prohibition and enforcement have certainly been successful: illicit-market cocaine costs 20 times the price of the licit pharmaceutical product, and much of the population has no easy access to the drug. But the capacity of more enforcement to drive prices higher, or even to prevent continued price declines, is very limited, as the drug law enforcement explosion of the past 15 years demonstrates. The value of enforcement in maintaining the borders between places where cocaine is easily available and places where it is not easily available is probably substantial, and it may well be that more enforcement at the margin will tend to slow the spread of the zone of easy availability, though that effect is hard to document. But of all users, the hard-core user/offenders are least likely to find themselves unable to acquire supplies.

Third, treatment. A wide variety of "modalities" have been shown to be effective in reducing drug consumption and criminal activity while the treatment lasts, seemingly regardless of whether entry into treatment is voluntary or coerced.[19] But even if there were sufficient treatment slots in programs appropriate to the criminal justice population, and even if treatment providers were motivated to serve user/offenders rather than other, less refractory clients, there would remain the problem of recruitment and retention. While some user/offenders want to quit, and even want to quit enough to go through the discomforts of the treatment process, many prefer, or act as if they prefer, cocaine or heroin, as long as they can get it.

In the abstract, there is a good case for expanding treatment capacity, focusing treatment on the user/offender population whose continued drug use imposes such high costs, and using the courts, prisons, and community corrections institutions to force user/offenders to enter, remain in, and comply with treatment. Adding drug treatment to incarceration makes sense, and good in-prison treatment with good post-release follow-up has been shown to reduce recidivism by about one-fifth,[20] thus more than paying for itself in budget terms alone.

But the unpopularity of user/offenders makes the funding problems difficult if not insoluble, the capacity and willingness of treatment providers to address the needs of this population remain unclear, and the administrative problems of enforcing treatment attendance and compliance through the criminal justice system are daunting. Starting from the current political situation and the current capacities and practices of the treatment system and the criminal justice system, it would be fatuous to expect expanded treatment availability to generate large changes in overall drug demand over the next several years.

So much for the repertoire of standard drug policies. Turning to corrections policies, we see a picture not much brighter. The routine functioning of the courts and corrections system does very little to address the substance abuse of those assigned to it, and much of that little is wrong.

Nominally, those on probation or parole are required to abstain from illegal activity, including drug possession, as a condition of their continued liberty. Almost all states give probation and parole officials the authority to administer drug tests, and a "dirty" (positive) test constitutes a violation of conditional release and thus grounds for sanctions, including revocation of conditional-release status and thus incarceration or re-incarceration, for a period up to the original nominal sentence.

In practice, however, most parole and (especially) probation offices are underfunded and overwhelmed by their caseloads; a big-city probation officer may be "managing" 150 offenders at any one time.[21] Funds for testing are scarce, and facilities for testing, including both equipment and staff to observe the specimen collection, even more so. If the specimens are sent out for analysis, turnaround time is measured in days. As a result, even special, "intensive supervision" probation efforts rarely test more than once a month,[22] and routine probation tests much less frequently than that. Thus a probationer on intensive supervision who uses cocaine or heroin has less than one chance in ten of being detected on any given occasion of use. (Perversely, marijuana is detectable for up to a month, making it the most likely to be detected.)

The result is widespread use, and therefore high rates of detection even with infrequent testing. That leaves the community corrections system in a bind. In most states, probation and parole officers have no individual power to sanction: they can only refer their wayward "clients" back to the parole board (for parolees) or the court (for probationers) with a recommendation that conditional-release status be revoked and the offender incarcerated or re-incarcerated. For probationers, the revocation hearing is a full adversarial proceeding; parole revocation is often simpler and usually swifter, but in any case there is a substantial paperwork burden. If the judge or parole board takes any action at all against the offender (by no means assured given the prison-crowding problem) it is likely to be severe: a few months behind bars is typical, and offenders have been sent back to finish multi-year sentences for a single positive marijuana test.

As a result, there are strong incentives, especially in the probation system, not to take every positive test back to the judge. Probationers may be counseled, warned, or referred to treatment providers several times before being (in the perhaps unintentionally graphic jargon term) "violated." It is hard to fault probation officers for attempting to "jawbone" their charges out of drug use rather than proceeding immediately to drastic measures. But the resulting system could hardly be more perverse in its effects.

An offender who has a strong craving for cocaine or heroin is put in a situation where the probability of detection conditional on one use is rather small, and the probability of punishment conditional on detection is larger, but still unknown and far less than certainty. For a hypothetical rational actor, the cumulative probability of eventually going to, or back to, prison for a period of months would be an ample deterrent: the "expected value" of the punishment is surely more than the user would willingly pay for the pleasure of a single evening with his favorite drug, and the randomness of the punishment would increase its disutility for anyone appropriately risk-averse. That is to say, the current system would be adequate—though still not optimal—to deter drug use by the sort of people who make and administer the laws.

Those who run afoul of the laws tend to behave differently. Crack-addicted burglars are much less likely to make careful comparisons between current benefits and anticipated future costs. Otherwise they would be neither crack-addicted nor burglars, since neither crack-smoking nor burglary is an activity with a net positive expected utility on any reasonable estimate of values and probabilities. The key to fixing the situation is to adapt the penalty structure to the decisionmaking styles of the people whose behavior one is trying to influence.[23]

Both casual empiricism and results from the psychology and behavioral-economics laboratories suggest that delay and uncertainty greatly weaken the effects of punishment, especially for those whose decisionmaking does not match the rational-actor models of textbook economics. Fitting deterrence regimes to the behavioral styles of hard-core user/offenders thus requires swift and certain, even if relatively mild, punishment rather than the current policy of randomized Draconianism.

Diversion and Drug Courts

Drug diversion and drug courts are the two major categories of special programs that attempt to use the authority of the criminal justice system to reduce drug use by offenders.[24]

Drug diversion involves offering a defendant the option of a deferred, suspended, or probationary sentence in lieu of possible incarceration on the condition of receiving drug substance abuse treatment. Diversion programs vary enormously. Some are formal treatment plans administered under the rubric of TASC (which once stood for "Treatment Alternatives to Street Crime" but now represents "Treatment Alternatives for Special Clients"), a network of specialists who find treatment placements for court-referred clients, monitor their progress, and report back to the court on treatment compliance. Others are as simple as a judge's demand for "30 in 30" (attendance at 30 12-Step meetings in the next 30 days) from someone accused of public intoxication or drunken driving.

In drug courts, the judge acts as the case manager rather than delegating that responsibility to a TASC provider. Defendants come in frequently to review their treatment compliance and drug-test results, and are praised or rebuked for good or bad conduct by the judge in open court. After a period of months, the defendant is sentenced on the original offense, with the promise that the sentence will reflect his presentencing behavior.

Because they are built around the idea of treatment, many diversion programs and drug courts tend to put as much stress on showing up for treatment sessions as they do on actual desistance from drug use. They vary widely in their use of immediate sanctions to enforce compliance. Some rely primarily either (for diversion programs) on the threat of removal from the program and sentencing on the original charge or (for drug courts) on the fact that sentencing is still to come.

Many drug court judges hope and believe that praise and reproof from the bench, backed with the judge's reserve powers of incarceration, will serve as sufficiently potent and immediate rewards and punishments without resorting to more material sanctions. Doubtless, they are right for some judges and some offenders.

What drug diversion and drug courts have in common is that participation is voluntary (defendants can, and some do, choose routine sentencing instead) and restricted to defendants whom the court and the prosecution are prepared *not* to incarcerate if the defendants will just clean up their acts. By their nature as "alternatives to incarceration," they cannot apply to those whose crimes have been especially severe. That excludes most violent crimes, and the federal law providing funding for drug courts specifies that defendants admitted to drug-court treatment must have no prior violent offenses either. Thus many of the most troublesome offenders, whose drug consumption it would be most valuable to influence, are excluded from the beginning.

Moreover, budget constraints limit drug-court and diversion populations; there is no mechanism by which the net cost savings they generate for the corrections system are recycled into program operations. Budgetary stringency both reinforces the programs' limited scope and creates a strong incentive for limited duration as well.

Typically, supervision under such programs lasts for periods measured in months: small fractions of typical addiction, and criminal, careers. This is not only a budgetary matter; it also derives from the limited leverage prosecutors have over most of the offenders eligible for diversion or drug-court processing. Offenders who refuse to enter these voluntary special programs and choose routine processing instead face relatively short prison or jail stays. In practice, some defendants prefer a short fixed period of incarceration to a longer period of supervision that may lead to incarceration if they backslide. The longer the period of supervision, the greater the incentive to just "do the time" and get it over with.

Thus limited scope and limited duration put an upper bound on the potential impact of diversion and drug courts. Making a larger impact could require a more comprehensive approach, embracing millions, rather than tens of thousands, of offenders and functioning as part of routine probation or parole supervision rather than as a special, voluntary program. Given current constraints on drug-treatment budgets, the requisite expansion in scale requires decoupling the testing-and-sanctions program from treatment, at least to the extent of imposing a requirement of abstinence on all drug-involved offenders, whether or not paid treatment slots are available for them.

Coerced Abstinence

To make a substantial dent in the drug consumption of addict/offenders, we need a system that will extend the supervisory capacities of drug courts and diversion programs to a larger proportion of the offender population and for longer periods. Such an approach would have to be simple enough to be operated successfully by ordinary judges and probation officers, rather than enthusiasts, cheap enough to be feasible from a budgetary standpoint, and sparing of scarce treatment and confinement capacity.

One option would be to substitute, to the maximum feasible extent, testing and automatic sanctions for services and personal attention from the judge. By contrast to coerced treatment, this approach might be called "coerced abstinence," because it aims directly at reduced drug consumption rather than at the intermediate goals of treatment entry, retention, and compliance.

Here's how such a system might work:

- Probationers and parolees are screened for cocaine, heroin, or methamphetamine use, using a combination of records review and chemical tests.
- Those identified as users, either at the beginning of their terms or by random testing thereafter, are subject to twice-weekly drug tests. They may choose any two days of the week and times of day for their tests, as long as the two chosen times are separated by at least 72 hours. That means that there is effectively no "safe window" for undetected use.
- Every positive test results in a brief (say, two-day) period of incarceration. (The length of the sanction, and whether and how sharply sanctions should increase with repeated violations, is a question best determined by trial and error, and the best answer

may vary from place to place. Maryland appears to be having good results with a program in which the first two "sanctions" are merely warnings. Where there exists a "community service"—that is, punitive labor—program with the capacity to enforce compliance, hours of work might make an excellent first sanction. Even for nonconfinement sanctions, confinement is needed as a backup threat for those who fail to comply.)

- The sanction is applied immediately, and no official has the authority to waive or modify it. (Perhaps employed users with no recent failures should be allowed to defer their confinement until the weekend to avoid the risk of losing their jobs.) The offender is entitled to a hearing only on the question of whether the test result is accurate; the penalty itself is fixed.
- Missed tests count as "dirty." (Perhaps the sanction should be somewhat greater, to discourage absconding.)
- After some long period (six months?) of no missed or positive tests, or alternatively achievement of some score on a point system, offenders are eligible for less frequent testing. Continued good conduct leads to removal to inactive status, with only random testing.

To operate successfully, such a program will require:

- the capacity to do tests at locations reasonably accessible to those being tested (since they have to appear twice a week);
- on-the-spot test results, both to shrink the time gap between misconduct and sanctions and to reduce the administrative burden of notifying violators and bringing them back for hearings and punishment;
- the capacity for quick-turnaround (within hours) verification tests on demand;
- authority to apply sanctions after an administrative hearing or the availability of an on-call judge who can hear a case immediately;
- confinement spaces for short-term detainees—or other sanctions capacity—available on demand; and
- the capacity to quickly apprehend those who fail to show up for testing.

None of these should be, in principle, impossible to obtain; but having all of them together, and reliably available, may well lie beyond the realm of practical possibility in many jurisdictions unless extraordinary political force is brought to bear. Thus elected officials will have to make coerced abstinence one of their goals, or it is unlikely to become a reality.

A wide variety of actual programs could be covered by the rubric "coerced abstinence." Crafting any particular implementation will require the resolution of several major design issues.

- One important but tricky decision involves what drugs to test for, both at the initial screen and for offenders under active monitoring. There is a strong case for omitting marijuana, at least at the initial screening stage: because it remains detectable for long periods and is widely used, any program that does not exclude it is likely to have a substantial proportion of marijuana-only clients. The individual and social benefits from reducing marijuana demand among offenders do not approach the benefits from reducing cocaine, methamphetamine, and heroin demand. On the other hand, once an offender is identified as a cocaine, methamphetamine, or heroin user, it may be that continued marijuana use will prove to be a risk factor for backsliding, both because it requires contact with drug sellers and because marijuana intoxication reduces sensitivity to the consequences of actions and thus deterrability. That suggests ignoring marijuana in the preliminary screening, but including it in ongoing monitoring.
- An especially touchy question is whether alcohol should be included. Its very short detection window makes it virtually impossible to detect all alcohol use, but very recent use is detectable in urine. Its legal status reduces the surface justification for forbidding it, but its link to violence (and complementarity with cocaine) creates a strong argument for doing so anyway. Alcohol could be another candidate for inclusion in routine testing but exclusion from the preliminary screening.
- The case for an automatic, and therefore necessarily formulaic, sanctions structure is very strong, and such a structure must start out with relatively mild sanctions or the program will col-

lapse of its own weight. But there is no analytic answer to the questions of how to start out and how rapidly, or how far, to increase severity with repeated violations; perhaps escalation will turn out to be unnecessary as long as some sanction is reliably delivered.

- Just as important as the sanctions structure is the reward structure: that rewards shape behavior more powerfully than punishments is well established. Of course, the political problems of rewarding lawbreakers for obeying the law are substantial ones, and the best feasible approach may be to use praise and reduced supervision as the primary forms of reward. But collecting an upfront "participation fee" or "fine" that is then returned in small increments for each "clean" test might greatly reduce the failure rate.
- After some period of compliance, both the need to reward desired behavior and simple budget pressures create a strong case for reduced supervision. Such crucial details as the schedule, the nature of the ongoing monitoring, and what to do with those who backslide under reduced supervision need to be resolved.
- Some participants will prove unable or unwilling to reform under punitive pressure alone. For that group, treatment is essential, if only to reduce the burden they put on sanctions capacity. In addition, it is probably true that the availability of treatment, or perhaps even a requirement to accept treatment, would cut down on violation rates. What sort of paid treatment to offer (and how to make use of the 12-Step programs), to whom it should be offered, and whether and under what circumstances it should be required, are all open questions.
- The crucial practical details of how to apprehend absconders and what sort of confinement capacity to maintain for violations need to be addressed.

Benefits and Costs

The costs and benefits of such programs will depend on details of their implementation, on local conditions, and on the (as yet largely unknown) behavior of offenders assigned to them. High compliance will translate into great benefits and modest costs, low compliance into the reverse. Only experience, ideally in the form of well-designed experiments, will allow informed judgments about whether, where, and how to put the concept of coerced abstinence into practice.

Still, it is possible to calculate in advance some of the costs and benefits of such programs under specified assumptions about design and results. Those calculations support the idea that coerced abstinence deserves a thorough set of trials.

Benefits

The catalogue of potential benefits is impressive. The primary benefit would be reduced drug abuse (to the extent that substitution is not complete), due not only to the deterrent effect of the sanctions but also to the "tourniquet" effect of interfering with incipient relapses before they can turn into full-fledged "runs" of heavy use. In the District of Columbia Drug Court experiment (see below) coercion outperformed (admittedly not very good) treatment.[25] That would suggest that successful coercion programs might match the reduction of two-thirds in drug consumption typical of users under treatment.

If that were right, and if all the high-dose user/offenders were under testing and sanctions, and if they account for 60 percent of total hard-drug consumption, the result would be a reduction in dealers' revenues of 40 percent. No other feasible anti-drug program offers any real hope of comparable levels of market shrinkage.

Smaller markets would have manifold benefits: shrinking access for potential new users, protecting neighborhoods from the side effects of illicit markets (most notably violence), diverting fewer adolescents and young adults away from school or licit work into dealing, and reduced diversion of police effort into drug law enforcement and prison capacity into holding convicted dealers. (Currently, about one-quarter of prison cells are occupied by persons serving sentences for drug dealing offenses;[26] shrinking that number by 40 percent would allow either a 10 percent cut in prison spending, for a savings of about $3.5 billion per year,[27] or increased imprisonment for nondealing offenses.)

The direct benefits of reduced consumption are comparably diverse: improved health; improved social functioning (job, family, neighborhood); and reduced crime by the offenders subject to testing and therefore reduced imprisonment demand among a population with a tendency to cycle in and out of confinement. With drug-involved offenders committing about half of all the felonies in big cities,[28] these potential benefits are great, though it would not be reasonable to expect a shrinkage in crime proportionate to the shrinkage in drug consumption. But if the reduction in overall offending were even half as large as the reduction in drug consumption, and if the sort of drug-involved offenders who would be subject to coerced abstinence account for 40 percent of the population behind bars for other than drug-dealing offenses, that would be another 13 percent of total confinement capacity (costing about $4 billion per year) saved, giving states the choice between increased deterrence and incapacitation for other offenders and cuts in prison spending.

A reliably operating coerced-abstinence system as part of probation and parole would also be expected to change the behavior of judges and parole boards with respect to making confinement decisions. By making probation and parole more meaningful alternatives to incarceration, the coerced-abstinence approach should lead to more use of community corrections in otherwise borderline cases. Instead of having to guess about whether a given drug-involved offender will elect to go straight this time, the decisionmaker can allow the offender to select himself for conditional freedom or confinement by his drug-taking behavior as revealed by the tests.

Coerced abstinence would also be expected to have beneficial effects on the treatment system. Some of those now referred to treatment by the courts would show themselves capable of abstaining from drug use without treatment, under the steady pressure of testing and sanctions, perhaps with the aid of a 12-Step fellowship or similar self-help group. Those in treatment would have increased incentive to succeed, with the pressure coming not from the therapist or the program but from an external force. Those not in treatment who found themselves incapable of complying on their own would have a strong incentive to find treatment, and their repeated failure would bring their need for treatment to the attention of the courts and community-corrections authorities, while the cost of their continual short confinement stays would create a financial incentive for the local government to provide it.

Costs

The cost picture is somewhat simpler, though still quite speculative until there are some working models to study. The important elements of cost would be testing operations, probation or parole supervision, sanctions and arrest capacity, and treatment, and a cost calculation will require both unit-cost and volume estimates. For unit costs, we can assume:

- Community-corrections officers at $60,000 per year, including fringe benefits, overhead, and supervision. Police officers at $100,000 per year, also inclusive.
- Testing at $5 for a five-drug screen. This is less than most agencies currently pay, but consistent with the current costs in the mass-production D.C. Pretrial Services Agency and not hard to imagine given the testing volumes that would exist with a full-scale national coerced-abstinence program.
- Confinement costs of $50/day, less than a typical jail, but consistent with the reduced need for services and security for short-term confinement: roughly the cost of a mediocre motel room.
- Treatment at $5,000 per year, reflecting a blend of methadone, outpatient drug-free counseling, and therapeutic communities for the most intractable. (Partly a design decision.)

In terms of volume, we can assume:

- 10 percent of the test results will be positive or no-shows. (This should be realistic for early stages of the program, perhaps pessimistic once the reliability of the tests and sanctions has been established in the minds of participants.)
- The average sanction for a violation is three days.
- 10 percent of active cases will be in mandated (paid) treatment, over and above those who would have been in treatment in the absence of the program. (Pure guess, and partly a design decision.)
- One-quarter of the population that originally qualified for active testing will have complied to the point of being moved to some form of low-cost monitoring and not been moved back to active

testing as a result of a violation. (Pure guess, and partly a design decision.)

- One probation or parole officer can manage 50 active testing-and-sanctions cases.
- One police officer to chase absconders is needed for each 250 active cases.

On these assumptions, total program costs for a group of 1,000 probationers who originally qualified for testing and sanctions, with 750 on active testing at any one time, would be as follows:

15 probation officers @ $60,000 = $0.9 million
3 police officers @ $100,000 = $0.3 million
750 offenders × 104 tests/year = 78,000 tests @ $5 = $0.4 million
78,000 tests × 10% × 3 days = 23,400 days @ $50 = $1.2 million
750 offenders × 10% = 75 treatment slots @ $5,000 = $0.4 million
TOTAL = $3.2 million; $3,200 per offender

This estimate of $3,200 per offender per year represents only about one-eighth of the annual cost of a prison cell. The probation department's share (probation salaries plus testing costs) would be $1,300 per offender, about twice the average annual cost of probation supervision.

Sources of Resistance

Anyone advocating a major change in the way a piece of the public's business is done must confront the public-sector version of the old question, "If yer so derned smart, why ain't ye rich?" If this is such a good idea, why is it not now being pursued? A variety of barriers, conceptual, organizational, and practical, have stood and still stand in the way of developing testing and sanctions into a working piece of administrative machinery.

Conceptually, the testing-and-sanctions approach challenges current understandings both of deterrence and of addiction. It seems hard to conceive that small sanctions would prove effective deterrents to those so signally resistant to the threat of large sanctions. (This resembles the question posed about bottle-deposit laws by the flacks for the beverage industries: "If a $500 fine doesn't stop a litterbug, what's a 5-cent deposit going to do?" The answer, of course, was that the $500 fine was largely notional, while the nickel actually gets collected.)

To some, the concept of addiction as a disease process involving loss of voluntary control over drug-taking implies that threats cannot change addictive behavior. This idea is related to the empirically discredited, but still powerful, notion that addiction implies that changes in price have little impact on the quantity purchased (inelastic demand).[29] There is laboratory-animal evidence that addictive demand is sensitive both to "price" (in the form of effort required) and to consequences[30] and human experimental evidence that immediate rewards for nonuse can substantially improve treatment success among those trying to quit.[31]

Since even pathological behaviors can be responsive to their consequences, the disease model of addiction does not rule out the possibility that coerced abstinence can succeed. Nonetheless, the notion that addicts are sick and therefore unresponsive to incentives remains a powerful one, and a strong source of resistance to testing-and-sanctions proposals.

In ideological terms, the testing-and-sanctions idea does not, at least at first blush, satisfy either the moralistic/punitive or the compassionate/therapeutic impulses that dominate the current political discourse about drugs, though it has something to offer to each side. That, plus its conceptual complexity, makes it unattractive as a political campaign proposal, except in the masquerade of yet another "get tough on drugs" proposal.

Alongside this lack of popular appeal is active unpopularity with an important interest group: treatment advocates. By no means do all treatment providers dislike coerced abstinence, but it encounters resistance among treatment administrators and advocates on three different grounds. Ideologically, it seems to be in tension with the disease concept of addiction, which is central to treatment providers' self-understanding and to their claims on public and private resources. In economic terms, coerced abstinence is one more competitor for scarce funds. (Curiously, some proponents of drug courts, who might also have been expected to see testing and sanctions as a competitor for funding, have instead been rather friendly toward the idea.) But at a deeper level, those with a strong commitment to drug treatment may reasonably regard testing and sanctions as an inferior substitute.

For some drug-involved offenders, simply getting rid of their drug habits would allow them to live substantially happier lives. But for many, their drug habits are only a part, and often the smaller part, of their problems. Drug treatment often involves addressing far more than drug problems; this is most evident in the case of therapeutic communities, with their holistic attempt to reshape character. From the viewpoint of those most concerned about persons with addictions, the testing-and-sanctions approach threatens to provide much, if not most, of the benefits of treatment from the viewpoint of crime victims and government budgets while providing little in the way of relief to those suffering from addiction.

The primary form this resistance has taken has been the attempt to redefine testing-and-sanctions proposals as programs either of coerced treatment or of treatment-needs assessment for the offender population. That process can be observed in the history of the Breaking the Cycle initiative, a joint effort of the National Institute of Justice and the Office of National Drug Control Policy.

Nor are the agencies most affected by coerced abstinence, and which will have to do most of the work, necessarily its supporters. Probation departments, usually badly overworked and understaffed, have not in general been aggressive in seeking out new missions and responsibilities. Police are anything but eager to make warrant service a high priority, though shifts toward community policing and toward holding area commanders responsible for reducing rates of criminal activity may be changing that. Corrections officials are not looking for new business, and especially not for the short-stay clients whose processing in and out takes so much effort.

Moreover, by contrast with ideas such as mandatory sentencing that are virtually self-implementing once legislation is passed, the degree of inter-agency coordination required to make a testing-and-sanctions program a success means that its implementation will require enormous effort on the part of whoever takes on the entrepreneurial role.

Finally, coerced abstinence suffers from two budget mismatches, one of timing and one of level of government. Even if the program turns out to be cost-neutral or better in the long run, there is no denying its immediate costs and immediate demands on scarce confinement capacity. The long-term savings are likely to be dismissed as typical program-advocate pie in the sky. Similarly, it is a rare county executive or sheriff who is eager to spend the county's resources on testing and sanctions in order to save the governor money in the form of reduced prison spending.

Experience

To date there are no hard published data about the effects of testing and sanctions on the model described above as part of routine probation and parole supervision in a large jurisdiction. Scattered judges have created such programs on their own initiative. Informal reports suggest good results, but there have been no published evaluations, and in any case such pioneer efforts often turn out to rely too heavily on the charismatic characteristics of their founders to be easily portable. There have been six more systematic efforts:

Santa Cruz County, California, instituted aggressive testing of known heroin users on probation in the late 1980s, along with a focused crackdown on street-level dealing. The county reported a 22 percent reduction in burglaries the following year, when burglaries were slightly up in adjacent comparable counties, but there was no careful examination of the relationship, if any, between the testing and the burglary reduction.

The Multnomah County, Oregon, Drug Testing and Evaluation Program looked like a testing-and-sanctions program at the outset, but evolved into merely one more tool in the probation officer's toolkit, with neither continuity of testing, predictability of sanctions, nor any real program integrity (in terms of which offenders were subject to it and which not). No firm conclusion could be drawn about its performance.

Project Sentry in Lansing, Michigan, has provided mostly short-term testing for drug-involved offenders on probation or presentencing release (about one-third of them felons) over the past 25 years. In the 29,650 specimens collected in the 15 months ended December 31, 1996, there were 3,096 positive tests (where each drug tested for counts as one test). If each positive test represented a different specimen, the positive rate per specimen would have been just over 10 percent; double-counting for multiple drugs detected from a single specimen would bring that figure down somewhat.[32]

The Connecticut Division of Parole has a few dozen parolees, identified before their release from prison as having had heroin or cocaine habits, on testing and sanctions, and reports very low rates (well under 5 percent) of positive tests. A new program will embrace a group of parolees who receive six-month reductions in their prison sentences in return for volunteering for 12 months of testing-and-sanctions coverage after release.

Maryland has the largest program to date, covering some 16,000 probationers.[33] Reportedly, the rate of "dirty" tests fell from about 40 percent when the program started to about 7 percent four months later. Like the Connecticut program, this cries out for formal evaluation.

The largest controlled trial to date has been the "sanctions track" of the District of Columbia Drug Court, where defendants randomly assigned to twice-a-week testing with immediate sanctions based on a formula took less drugs than either those mandated to treatment or those assigned to routine drug-court processing (with test results reviewed by a judge and considered at sentencing time). Since the D.C. drug court is not restricted to drug-defined offenses but includes drug-involved defendants facing a variety of charges, this result may have some application to the broader run of felony and misdemeanor offenders, but the fact that the drug court is a voluntary diversion program limits the inferences that can be drawn about the potential of testing and sanctions as an element of routine probation.[34]

The Breaking the Cycle program in Birmingham, Alabama, now operating with federal research funding, is intended to be a full-scale test combining testing and sanctions with treatment, and an elaborate evaluation is planned.

Experimental Approaches

Two sorts of experiments ought to be done to help define the feasibility and utility of testing-and-sanctions programs: one taking the offender as the unit of analysis, the other taking the jurisdiction. Given the variety of circumstances and possible program implementations, each type of experiment should probably be run in more than one location, and in each case a strong argument can be made for a shakedown period of trial-and-error program development before any formal evaluation starts. Too many promising innovations have run aground on the shoals of single, premature evaluations.

At the individual level, one would want to test the extent to which offenders made subject to a well-implemented testing-and-sanctions program would modify their drug-taking behavior and the effect of those modifications on crime and social functioning. That same test would provide estimates of failure rates and thus of sanctions demand. At its simplest, an experiment would involve the random assignment of offenders to either business-as-usual processing or testing and sanctions. A useful way to complicate such an experiment would be to introduce systematic variation within the testing-and-sanctions condition, to help answer some of the program-design questions.

Jurisdiction-level experiments would be, in effect, pilot implementations, with results compared either to "control" jurisdictions or to historical results. Either basis of comparison brings with it substantial methodological issues, but there are two sets of questions that can be answered only at the jurisdictional level:

- How closely can the actual performance of courts, probation, police, corrections, and treatment organizations approach to the theoretical design of a testing-and-sanctions program?
- What effect would such a program have on the local drug markets? Here the quantities of interest would include the level of dealing activity, the extent of market-related disorder and violence, and the numbers of dealing-related arrests, convictions, and sentences.

Recent Developments

Proposals for coerced abstinence started to float around in Clinton Administration circles almost from the beginning of the first Clinton term, but they were sidetracked into the more treatment-oriented Breaking the Cycle experiment and never emerged into political prominence. But during the run-up to the 1996 elections, coerced abstinence was adopted, first as an Administration proposal and then as a law requiring every state to create a program of testing and sanctions for drug-involved offenders as a condition of receiving federal grants to build prisons. Opponents of the program in the Justice Department managed to write the implementing regulations so as to restrict the requirements, even for planning, to prisoners and parolees, exempting the much larger number of probationers.

Still, every state now has to consider whether and how to make drug testing-and-sanctions abstinence a part of the criminal justice process. The current approach to drug-involved offenders makes so little sense from any perspective that something almost has to replace it. Perhaps that something will turn out to be some version of coerced abstinence.

Notes

I have been cultivating this set of ideas for more than a decade now, and a full list of my intellectual debts would be very long. Jerome Jaffe, John Kaplan, Robert DuPont, Eric Wish, and Jerry Gallegher all made theoretical and/or practical contributions to the offender-testing idea before I started working on it. A very special debt is owed to Will Brownsberger, who has been working hard to keep me honest about what is known and what is not known, what is practically possible and what isn't about this topic.

1. This is much smaller than the estimated number of persons "suffering from" or "in need of treatment for" substance abuse disorders. It excludes (1) those whose primary problem drug is nicotine or alcohol (not illicit); (2) those whose primary drug problem is cannabis (not very expensive, and only weakly connected to crime by users and violence and disorder among dealers); and those who support their expensive hard-drug habits without committing crimes for which they get repeatedly arrested (earning it, getting it as presents or as public income-support payments, spending savings or inheritances, or committing crimes but not getting caught).

2. Office of Applied Studies, *Preliminary Estimates from the 1995 National Household Survey on Drug Abuse* (Rockville, Md.: Substance Abuse and Mental Health Services Administration, Aug. 1996).

3. William Rhodes, Paul Scheiman, Tanutda Pittayathikhun, Laura Collins, and Vared Tsarfaty, *What America's Users Spend on Illegal Drugs, 1988–1993* (Washington: Office of National Drug Control Policy, 1995).

4. Office of Justice Programs, *1995 Drug Use Forecasting Annual Report on Adult and Juvenile Arrestees* (Washington: U.S. Department of Justice, 1996).
5. Peter Reuter, "Can We Make Prohibition Work Better? Assessing American Drug Policy," speech delivered in Washington, Feb. 11, 1997.
6. Bureau of the Census, *Statistical Abstract of the United States: 1998,* table 500.
7. Reuter, "Can We Make Prohibition Work Better?"
8. *Statistical Abstract of the United States: 1998,* 207.
9. Centers for Disease Control and Prevention, *U.S. HIV and AIDS Cases Reported through June 1996,* vol. 8, no. 1 (Atlanta: U.S. Department of Health and Human Services, 1996), table 3.
10. Reuter, "Can We Make Prohibition Work Better?"
11. Rhodes et al., *What America's Users Spend,* table 3.
12. Norris O. Johnson, "The Pareto Law," *Review of Economics and Statistics,* Feb. 1937, 20; D. H. Macgregor, "Pareto's Law," *Economic Journal,* March 1936, 80.
13. Office of Applied Studies, *Preliminary Estimates;* Reuter, "Can We Make Prohibition Work Better?"
14. Rhodes et al., *What America's Users Spend,* table 3.
15. Ibid., 10.
16. William Rhodes, "Synthetic Estimation Applied to the Prevalence of Drug Use," *Journal of Drug Issues* 23, no. 2 (1993): 297–321.
17. Some cutting-edge programs have shown substantial value in preventing initiation to hard-drug use among high-risk populations—but those are not the programs getting the bulk of current funding. See Jonathan Caulkins et al., *An Ounce of Prevention, A Pound of Uncertainty: The Cost-Effectiveness of School-Based Drug Prevention Programs* (Santa Monica: Rand, 1999).
18. Mark A. R. Kleiman, "Reducing the Prevalence of Cocaine and Heroin Dealing among Adolescents," *Valparaiso University Law Review* 31, no. 2 (May 1997): 551–564.
19. Carl G. Leukefeld and Frank M. Tims, *Compulsory Treatment of Drug Abuse: Research and Clinical Practice,* NIDA Research Monograph 86, National Institute on Drug Abuse, 1988.
20. Harry Wexler, Douglas Lipton, and K. Forester, "Outcome Evaluation of a Prison Therapeutic Community for Substance Abuse Treatment," *Criminal Justice Behavior* 17, no. 1 (March 1990): 71–92.
21. Bureau of Justice Statistics, *Sourcebook of Criminal Justice Statistics—1994* (Washington: Department of Justice, 1995), table 1.71.
22. Joan Petersilia and Susan Turner, "Intensive Probation and Parole," and Joan Petersilia, "Probation in the United States," in Michael Tonry, ed., *Crime and Justice: An Annual Evaluation of Research,* vol. 17 (Chicago: University of Chicago Press, 1993). Mark A. R. Kleiman, "Community

Corrections as the Front Line in Crime Control," *UCLA Law Review* 46, no. 6 (Aug. 1999).

23. Mark A. R. Kleiman, "Getting Deterrence Right: Applying Tipping Models and Behavioral Economics to the Problems of Crime Control," in *Perspectives on Crime and Justice, 1999* (Washington: National Institute of Justice, forthcoming).

24. On drug courts see Adele Harrell, *Drug Courts and the Role of Graduated Sanctions* (Washington: National Institute of Justice, 1998); National Association of Drug Court Professionals, Drug Court Standards Committee, *Defining Drug Courts: The Key Components* (Washington: U.S. Department of Justice, Office of Justice Programs, 1997); Drug Court Clearinghouse and Technical Assistance Project at American University, *Looking at a Decade of Drug Courts* (Washington: U.S. Department of Justice, Office of Justice Programs, 1998).

25. Adele Harrell and Shannon Cavanagh, *Preliminary Results from the Evaluation of the D.C. Superior Drug Intervention Program for Drug Felony Defendants* (Washington: Urban Institute, 1997).

26. Reuter, "Can We Make Prohibition Work Better?"

27. Bureau of Justice Statistics, *Sourcebook,* table 1.3.

28. Office of Justice Programs, *1995 Drug Use Forecasting Annual Report on Adult and Juvenile Arrestees* (Washington: U.S. Department of Justice, 1996).

29. Jonathan P. Caulkins, "Estimating the Elasticity of Demand for Cocaine and Heroin," manuscript, Carnegie Mellon University.

30. Gene M. Heyman, "Resolving Contradictions of Addiction," *Behavioral and Brain Sciences* 19 (1995); Mark Kleiman, "Addiction, Rationality, Behavior and Measures: Some Comments on the Problems of Integrating Econometric and Behavioral Economic Research," in Frank J. Chaloupka et al., eds., *The Economic Analysis of Substance Use and Abuse: An Integration of Econometric and Behavioral Economic Research* (Chicago: University of Chicago Press, 1999). Also in Chaloupka et al., Stephen Higgins, "Applying Behavioral Economics to the Challenge of Reducing Cocaine Abuse," and Nancy M. Petry and Warren K. Bickel, "A Behavioral Economic Analysis of Polydrug Abuse in Heroin Addicts."

31. S. T. Higgins, A. J. Budney, W. K. Bickel, F. E. Foerg, R. Donham, and G. J. Badger, "Incentives Improve Outcome in Outpatient Behavioral Treatment of Cocaine Dependence," *Archives of General Psychiatry* 51 (1994): 568–576.

32. J. J. Gallegher, "Project Sentry Final Program Report" (Lansing, Mich.: Project Sentry, 1996).

33. See Faye S. Taxman, *Task Force on Drug-Addicted Offenders* (Office of the Lieutenant Governor of Maryland, 1997).

34. Harrell and Cavanagh, *Preliminary Results.*

Limits on the Role of Testing and Sanctions   **7**

William N. Brownsberger

The control of substance abuse among those already involved with the criminal justice system should be a fundamental component of our anti-drug strategy. However, local patterns of drug use and criminal offending should influence the targeting and structure of testing-and-sanctions programs. In many areas, we should implement testing and sanctions primarily in conjunction with drug treatment and primarily for persons who are both heavily addicted and charged with serious offenses.

Role of Testing and Sanctions in Assessment

Prosecutors, judges, and defense attorneys tend to settle cases with an implicit view of an appropriate escalation of sanctions in which the first few offenses receive modest responses. This practice is understandable: the vast majority of offenses are, in fact, relatively minor, and most offenders never progress to more serious crime.[1] However, this approach is inadequate for the subgroup of offenders who, although perhaps corrigible, are given enough rope to hang themselves—are allowed to progress with impunity until they earn a debilitating long incarceration.

It is very difficult to make an early identification of offenders likely to repeat their offenses. The best scientific assessment models using information typically available to criminal justice decisionmakers can explain only a small portion of the variance in recidivism.[2] To some extent this uncertainty may be irreducible, as it may reflect the picaresque nature of the criminal career—the criminal may be pulled into or out of delinquency by a variety of unpredictable external influences. On the other hand, prediction may be somewhat improved with more information. A major emerging strategy turns on greater involvement of other community service agencies and the community itself in identifying troublesome defendants. Drug testing is, perhaps, the only other new source of information for improving the identification of high-risk offenders.

In order to understand the limited role of drug testing in identifying likely recidivists, it is helpful to understand more clearly what is known about the relationship between drug use and crime. A majority of illegal drug users are *not* otherwise delinquent, and many more of them, even though otherwise delinquent, are not the highly destructive recidivists we are most concerned to identify and address. Marijuana use and even occasional use of hard drugs (cocaine or heroin) has, for several decades, been far more widespread than predatory delinquency.[3] Even among frequent users of hard drugs, many are relatively moderate users and relatively low-rate offenders. Studies of frequent cocaine users have suggested that some use over one gram per day.[4] One million users consuming one gram per day would annually consume more cocaine than is successfully imported into the United States.[5] Yet the cocaine frequent-user population is estimated at about 2 million.[6] Similarly, reported crime rates in *some* frequent-user populations are so high that if extended across all frequent users they would account for an order of magnitude more crimes than are actually committed.[7]

For the user/offenders whose drug use and criminal offending are both at relatively moderate levels, there is no reason to assume that their offending is *caused* by their use. Longitudinal studies have made clear that, when both are present, the onset of delinquency in adolescence is more likely to precede the onset of drug use than the reverse. By contrast, for truly heavy drug users, that is, users who use many times every day, it is clear that their high-cost habits drive high rates of property crime. In street drug-user populations, those admitting higher current levels of use admit higher current frequencies of offending. Similarly, in prison populations, those admitting higher historical levels of use admit higher historical frequencies of offending. In populations undergoing drug treatment, offending frequencies fall as drug use falls.[8]

With this perspective, we can return to the question of how to use drug testing in predicting recidivism. From a recidivism-prevention standpoint, the greatest benefits come from the identification of truly heavy users. A dirty random test does not necessarily identify a truly heavy user or a prospective truly heavy user. Nor do a few clean tests rule out the possibility of truly heavy use—some addicts do "go on the wagon." Similarly, if there is no reliable sanction consequent to a dirty test, the frequent but non-addicted user may simply continue to use, and even a string of dirty tests may not indicate a hard-core addict or a likely high-rate offender.

Mark A. R. Kleiman's coerced-abstinence regime, in which frequent testing is combined with annoying sanctions for dirty tests, may be an effective approach to identifying heavy users. The offender who fails repeatedly in a coerced-abstinence regime is likely to be an addicted truly heavy user and so a likely future recidivist. However, the use of coerced abstinence as a screening tool is probably rarely warranted. The costs of the tool go beyond the few hundred dollars it would cost on average per offender to test and sanction the mostly non-addicted universe of all offenders during a screening period. Requiring light offenders to appear for frequent drug testing may, in itself, constitute a significant increase in punishment. If they test dirty and end up in jail, the increment will be even greater, and of course, they will be brought into closer contact with more hardened offenders. Many will be less willing to plead guilty and avoid trial. The predisposition litigation costs of imposing the increased intrusion of drug testing and sanctions would be significant. In jurisdictions where heavy substance abuse is less common, the costs of the screen would be almost entirely an increase in both short- and long-run costs, offset only by rare addict-detection benefits.

A coerced-abstinence screening program limited to serious offenders is more likely to be cost-justifiable. These offenders are facing a more stringent punishment, and the intrusion of frequent drug testing is thus relatively less significant in the plea bargaining process, so that the change in pre-disposition costs would be less. More of these offenders are likely to turn out to be addicted, and the cost of screening is more likely to be amortized by increased detection. Yet even here one may ask whether a coerced-abstinence screening program will pay for itself in increased accuracy of detection over interviews, observations, and consultation with community partners. There are no data that illuminate this precise question, but careful empirical analysis indicates that less systematic drug testing adds little predictive power to traditional assessment tools.[9] The cost-benefit ratio depends not only on the skills and resources of assessment staff but also on the local epidemiology of substance abuse. Only where, as a result of both high prevalence and unsuccessful detection, a good deal of substance abuse is going undetected with the existing tools is wide use of coerced abstinence likely to be warranted *as a detection tool.*

Technology in the testing area is evolving rapidly toward lower costs, quicker results, more specificity about the quantity and recency of use, detection of more drugs, and greater accuracy. New systems for installation in the offender's home are making alcohol monitoring more feasible. Information systems for reporting and interpreting test history are also improving.[10] All of these trends may make testing, either random or in a coerced-abstinence program, more consistently cost-justifiable as a screening tool over the years to come. However, since testing without sanctions may be counterproductive and imposing sanctions is costly, most jurisdictions will have to continue to experiment in order to determine the optimal scope of testing for screening purposes.

Role of Testing and Sanctions in Intervention Strategies

For those offenders identified as high-risk and in need of intervention, either through their records, through community and agency input, or through a coerced-abstinence screening program, many new interventions are emerging which do not involve long-term incarceration, and which can be applied early in an offender's career, perhaps preventing him from progressing to incarceration.[11] These interventions defy easy classification, and it is too soon to embrace them without reservation. The key themes are to reach more deeply into the offender's life—to monitor him more closely, to protect him from criminogenic influences, to offer him the rehabilitative programming he may need, and to offer more immediate positive and negative motivations to good behavior.

For the non-addicted but otherwise high-risk user/offender who is allowed to remain on the street, testing and sanctions are best seen as possible components of an overall regime of intense supervision. A positive drug test may be taken as an indicator that the offender is moving again in the wrong circles and is likely to be drawn into other forms of delinquency. Used in conjunction with bed-checking visits to verify curfews, street contact in partnership with police, and other proactive supervision approaches, drug testing intensifies the pressure on the offender to choose a non-delinquent lifestyle. But the drug testing, however frequent and however combined with sanctions, may not be the most important element of the overall intervention. If the offender has stopped smoking crack or chipping heroin, but still runs with the same dangerous crowd, perhaps drinking heavily while complaining noisily about the twice-weekly drug testing, his risk of recidivism may be not at all diminished.

For the addicted offender, drug testing and sanctions have a more central role, but other forms of intervention may also be essential. The modest sanctions contemplated in coerced abstinence may, in themselves, have little power to influence addicts' behavior. Most addicted users of hard drugs are unemployable and yet need to generate a significant income. They accept enormous risks and actual negative consequences daily to maintain their habit. They commit a variety of income-producing crimes with varying apprehension and violence risks. They steal from dealers who punish them corporally. They prostitute themselves. They use street drugs that may be fatally potent or contain fatal adulterants. They end up in the emergency room repeatedly. And of course, if they have a family, social, or economic life to ruin, they ruin it quickly. It is unrealistic to expect that the threat of a weekend or a week or a year in jail would make a large alteration in their decisionmaking calculus. This should seem unrealistic even to theorists who reject the received definition of addiction, which turns on the concept of a subjective loss of ability to control use in the face of negative consequences.

As to these truly heavy users, coerced abstinence by itself is likely to have, at best, second-order benefits: the heavy users' repeated failures and re-incarcerations may help "bottom them out" and drive them into detoxification and treatment. Their failures may also make it easier for the criminal justice system to incarcerate them and incapacitate them as offenders. In the context of treatment, testing and sanctions may help break through denial and deception. For truly heavy users, coerced abstinence should be seen not as a stand-alone control strategy as Kleiman suggests, but as an important adjunct to the existing strategies of treatment and incarceration.

Between light, non-criminogenic use and truly heavy use, there is a continuum of use levels which correlates with a continuum of dependence, a continuum of personal harm, and a continuum of criminal-offending rates. It seems likely that in the middle area there is a group whose drug use and drug-use-related offending are both significant yet both possibly responsive to the pressure of a coerced-abstinence regime alone. This group may include some offenders on a down-slope into addiction and high-rate offending. If one believes that this middle group is large, then one may want to implement coerced abstinence on a broad scale, perhaps for all offenders who commit offenses above a fixed level of seriousness, without attempting to limit application to the heaviest users. Significant reductions in demand and offending might accrue. If, on the other hand, one believes that the offender population is skewed toward the two ends of the use-level continuum, one may see coerced abstinence as having a much more limited role.

The size of the middle group has to vary across localities and subpopulations. Cultural patterns of controlled drug use may sometimes allow high prevalence of moderate use with relatively little criminogenic effect. Cultural patterns of uncontrolled use may tend to make use more likely to cause criminality and may tend to create a broad middle group of user/offenders. Temporal patterns of the emergence of epidemics may also affect the shape of the use-level distribution. As epidemics are expanding, there may be a large group of users midway down the slope to addiction; coerced abstinence may be very helpful at this stage. When epidemics have stabilized, the population may be more clearly divided between light controlled users and addicts. Given the great difficulty of collecting reliable data on heavy drug use and criminal offending patterns even locally and given the difficulty of generalization it seems clear that the size of the middle group will permanently remain an imponderable at the national level. Advocacy of coerced abstinence should be accordingly qualified.

Additional Implementation Considerations

The marginal benefit-cost ratio of testing and sanctions as against other components of an integrated response to addiction (or to non-addictive abuse) remains very unclear. Kleiman computes the cost of a coerced-abstinence program as $3,200 per offender per year. However, this represents an average in a universal application of the program. For the core of truly heavy users, the costs for testing and sanctions are much higher.[12] High-intensity testing will need to be maintained longer. The dirty-test and no-show rates will be much higher, and the apprehension and incarceration costs will accordingly increase dramatically. The testing-and-sanctions program may be far more expensive than court-supervised outpatient treatment, even including intermittent residential detoxification, especially if the outpatient treatment takes the almost cost-free form of a mandated 12-Step program in a court facility. In some instances the in-and-out-of-jail churning associated with coerced abstinence may be more expensive than simple incarceration.

Since coerced abstinence relies heavily on punishment, there are affirmative reasons to avoid implementing it on a stand-alone basis. A pure strategy of testing and punishment runs the risk over time of creating an expensive backlash. Sanctions aside, drug testing involves the degrading tedium of frequent court visits and is in itself humiliating since the officer taking the sample must observe the production of the sample. If the testing and sanctions are administered as part of a treatment program and/or under the supervision of a drug court judge, the addicts are much more likely to understand them as well-intended. For the down-and-out criminal addict whose street environment is very bleak, a small dose of support and encouragement may have much stronger positive effect than a large dose of punishment.[13]

Our criminal justice system is an adversary system but works primarily through accommodations among adversaries. New rules that are not carefully negotiated and marketed to all players run into enormous friction. To the extent that defense counsel do not accept the concept of testing with sanctions as positive for their clients, they can assert procedural rights which will defeat the increased certainty of sanctioning. The high transaction costs associated with the imposition of sanctions are a major reason for the usual counterproductive approach to probation and parole surrenders—tolerance of many small violations until they amount to a large violation meriting an extended incarceration. Any jurisdiction seeking to expand the use of drug testing with sanctions must take an inclusive approach to the planning process with the goal of recruiting the defense bar in support of an appropriately balanced regime.

Kleiman rightly points to the critical role of police in making a testing-and-sanctions program work. The best-run police departments have realized by now that warrant service is a very important crime-control tool. High-risk offenders who have defaulted on an obligation to the court (any obligation, but especially the obligation to take a drug test) are very likely to be current high-rate offenders. An emphasis on testing and sanctions, provided it is appropriately focused on high-risk offenders, is very consistent with community policing priorities. On the other hand, an overly broad program that requires police to chase many low-priority offenders is unlikely to win police support for warrant service.

Kleiman argues for an absolutely rigid approach to the application of sanctions. He makes the very valid point that if the schedule is absolutely rigid, then, in a perversely liberating sense, responsibility is placed on the addict for compliance. Yet addicts often make poor decisions with adverse consequences not only for themselves but for others (such as children under their care). Some flexibility as to the type and timing of punishment administered for a dirty test may be needed to protect addicts and their dependents from their mistakes. There is no empirical reason to believe that the marginally reduced certainty of punishment resulting from judicious exercise of discretion will make the difference between renewed abstinence and uncontrolled relapse. It is a fantasy to believe that the system can create absolute certainty of response anyway—addicts can always hope to beat the test and often do except in the best-run programs,[14] and, of course, they can always abscond and apprehension is necessarily uncertain.

The issue of continuity remains the most difficult problem to solve. There is no reason to expect that a successful period of coerced abstinence will be followed by continued abstinence once probation or parole ends. In fact, there may be a sharp rebound when coerced abstinence is ended. While no such rebound effect has been associated with treatment (which usually seeks to teach the addict how to abstain and why to want to abstain), long-term follow-up of addicts usually indicates eventual relapse.[15] Addicts, treated or untreated, are as likely to die in any given year as they are to achieve stable abstinence. The course of addiction to heroin, cocaine, or alcohol may run for decades. Coerced abstinence, like treatment, will probably pay for itself on the day it is administered (provided it is administered to a truly heavy user whose use reduction will materially benefit the public).[16] Yet, to truly protect the public (and to help drug users recover) we need to develop regimes under which monitoring can be continued for longer periods.

Summary

In summary, in my view, coerced abstinence, as defined by Kleiman, should not be understood as a universal program. It has four possible roles: A brief regime can serve as a systematic method for identification of addicts, but in many jurisdictions the incremental detection benefits may not be worth the cost. A regime of varying intensity (perhaps below Kleiman's twice-weekly prescription) can serve as part of a generally intense community supervision program for non-addict offenders who have been identified as high-risk for reasons other than their drug use. A heavy testing schedule, probably with sanctions, is an essential concomitant of treatment and aftercare for addicted truly heavy users. A heavy testing schedule with sanctions may have significant stand-alone crime-control value for medium-level users, but the size of this group is unclear.

It is particularly questionable to characterize coerced abstinence as a stand-alone demand-reduction strategy. Most analysts agree that the 2 million "heavy" users of cocaine account for a large share of the cocaine demand. In this computation, however, the term "heavy" refers to those using weekly or more often. This is very different from our use of the term "heavy" as applied to our national drug of choice, alcohol. Although good statistics are nonexistent, in light of the arguments in the preceding section it is reasonable to believe that a few hundred thousand addicted truly heavy users of cocaine and heroin, who use many times a day, account for most the cocaine and heroin consumed. On the one hand, these users may not respond to testing and sanctions. On the other hand, reducing or even ending use by the other weekly users—light and medium-level users who may respond to a testing-and-sanctions regime—may make only a very modest dent in overall demand.

Notes

1. See, e.g., Massachusetts Sentencing Commission, *Report to the General Court* (Boston, 1996), which includes a study of the sentences received by all persons convicted in Massachusetts criminal courts in fiscal 1994. Offenses at seriousness levels 1–3 (of 9 levels) accounted for 90 percent of all offenses. The first two levels consist primarily of misdemeanors. The third level includes, for example, assault and battery with a dangerous weapon resulting in no or minor injury and larcenies under $10,000. Moreover, there is a larger universe of persons (unmeasured in the Sentencing Commission Report which only examines convictions) who are charged with and guilty of provable minor offenses but whose cases are dismissed with a warning, perhaps on payment of court costs.

   Offenders with no record or under six offenses at the bottom two levels of seriousness ("no/minor" records) account for over half (51.7 percent) of the convictions. From this, it follows that the "no/minor" record group includes a large number of offenders who encounter much less than annually or will never again encounter the criminal justice system. In a world in which most offenders continued to offend regularly, those at the early stages of long offending careers would necessarily constitute a very small share of the case flow.

2. See Peter R. Jones, "Risk Prediction in Criminal Justice," and James Bonta, "Risk-Needs Assessment and Treatment," in A. Harland, ed., *Choosing Correctional Options That Work* (Thousand Oaks, Calif.: Sage, 1996).

3. The 1996 National Household Survey on Drug Abuse indicated that 13.0 million *persons* nationwide would have admitted past-month use of an illegal drug, and 5.8 million would have admitted use of a drug other than

marijuana. See www.health.org/pubs/nhsda/96hhs/rtst1002g.htm. Despite recent increases, this is a historically low level. The total number of violent and property *crimes* known to police in 1994 was 14.0 million, of which only 1.9 million were violent. This is a historically high level despite recent decreases. See Kathleen Maguire and Ann L. Pastore, eds., *Sourcebook of Criminal Justice Statistics, 1995* (Washington: Bureau of Justice Statistics, 1996), tables 3.109–3.110. Given that many offenders commit many crimes annually—see Jan M. Chaiken and Marcia R. Chaiken, "Drugs and Predatory Crime," in Michael R. Tonry and James Q. Wilson, eds., *Drugs and Crime* (Chicago: University of Chicago Press, 1990)—it is clear that the universe of serious current offenders was considerably smaller than the universe of current drug users, even in the mid-1990s, a relatively low-drug-use, high-crime era.

4. The national surveys do not effectively reach frequent users. See William Rhodes, "Synthetic Estimation Applied to the Prevalence of Cocaine Use," *Journal of Drug Issues* 23, no. 2 (1993): 297–321; and William Brownsberger, "Prevalence of Frequent Cocaine Use in Urban Poverty Areas," *Contemporary Drug Problems* 24, no. 2 (1997): 349–371. Our knowledge of the characteristics of heavy-user populations is sketchy and derives primarily from ethnographic and statistical studies of local populations, often in treatment or in prison. Data points suggesting usage well over one gram per day by the right tail of the right tail of the use-level distribution include B. Edlin et al., "Intersecting Epidemics—Crack Cocaine Use and HIV Infection among Inner-City Young Adults," *New England Journal of Medicine* 331 (1994): 1422–27 (nonrepresentative street sample of inner-city crack users used a *median* of 28 days in the last month and a *median* of 10 times per day; at 0.1 grams per use, this would translate roughly into a *median* consumption of 340 grams per year); R. Booth, J. Watters, and D. Chitwood, "HIV Risk-Related Sex Behaviors among Injection Drug Users, Crack Smokers and Injection Drug Users Who Smoke Crack," *American Journal of Public Health* 83 (1993): 1144–48 (significant share of sample of mixed drug users reported over 250 occasions of use within the past 30 days); Peter Reuter, Robert MacCoun, and Patrick Murphy, *Money from Crime: A Study of the Economics of Drug Dealing in Washington, D.C.* (Santa Monica: Rand, 1990) (estimates *mean* monthly expenditure of Washington, D.C., dealers who admit spending for drugs for their own use of $1,596, suggesting *mean* consumption well over 200 grams per year, or more if the dealers are supplying themselves at wholesale rates under $100 per gram); and M. Rattner, ed., *Crack Pipe as Pimp: An Ethnographic Investigation of Sex-for-Crack Exchanges* (New York: Lexington Books, 1992) (six studies of crack use and sexual behavior indicating difficulty of measuring usage by crack addicts but consistent with usage over one gram per day during binges).

5. Total un-interdicted cocaine importation into the United States is on the order of 300 million grams per year. See, e.g., Susan S. Everingham and C. Peter Rydell, *Modeling the Demand for Cocaine* (Santa Monica: Rand, 1994).

6. See Rhodes, "Synthetic Estimation."

7. Rhodes (ibid.) estimates roughly 600,000 weekly heroin users in the United States. Several populations of heroin-addicted prison inmates estimated their own pre-incarceration annual robbery rates at between 5 and 35; see Chaiken and Chaiken, "Drugs and Predatory Crime." If all heroin addicts were equally heavy users and equally high-rate offenders, one would expect millions of robberies per year by them alone, while the actual number of robberies known to the police nationwide was only 618,000 in 1994; see Maguire and Pastore, *Sourcebook*.

8. See Chaiken and Chaiken, "Drugs and Predatory Crime."

9. William Rhodes, Raymond Hyatt, and Paul Scheiman, "Predicting Pretrial Misconduct with Drug Tests of Arrestees: Evidence from Eight Settings," *Journal of Quantitative Criminology* 12, no. 3 (1996): 315–348. This study leaves open the possibility that a positive test for heroin, as opposed to cocaine, may in fact have some predictive power.

10. See, e.g., John A. Carver, Kathryn R. Boyer, and Ronald Hickey, "Management Information Systems and Drug Courts: The District of Columbia Approach," paper prepared for the 1995 National Symposium on the Implementation and Operation of Drug Courts.

11. See generally Harland, *Choosing Correctional Options*.

12. Of course, the benefits of testing and sanctions of the truly heavy users may be higher too. Jonathan Caulkins (private communication) has computed that even at an average of $3,200 per offender the benefit of expenditure on coerced abstinence is considerably less than the benefit of treating heavy users. Caulkins computes the reduction in cocaine consumed for every $1 million spent on treatment as 103.6 kg. Using the same measurement framework, the reduced consumption works out to 29.1 kg per $1 million spent on coerced abstinence, following Kleiman's assumption of a 2/3 reduction in consumption for each heavy user in the program. This computation is subject to a number of challenges; most important, David Boyum points out that treatment is assumed to have future-year benefits in Caulkins's analysis while coerced abstinence is not. At best, one can conclude that the cost-benefit comparison of coerced abstinence to treatment is uncertain. On drug-testing programs see Francis Cullen, J. Wright, and Brandon Applegate, "Control in the Community: The Limits of Reform?" in Harland, *Choosing Correctional Options*.

13. See, e.g., Paul Gendreau, "The Principles of Effective Intervention with Offenders," in Harland, *Choosing Correctional Options*.

14. See Sam Torres, "The Use of a Credible Drug Testing Program for Accountability and Intervention," *Federal Probation* 60, no. 4 (1996): 18–23.

15. See George E. Vaillant, *The Natural History of Alcoholism Revisited* (Cambridge, Mass.: Harvard University Press, 1995); Vaillant, "Twelve-Year Follow-up of New York Narcotic Addicts, II: The Natural History of a Chronic Disease," *New England Journal of Medicine* 275, no. 23 (1966): 1282–88.

16. On the payback of investments in treatment see, e.g., Dean R. Gerstein, Robert A. Johnson, Henrick J. Harwood, Douglas Fountain, Natalie Suter, and Kathryn Malloy, "Evaluating Recovery Services: The California Drug and Alcohol Assessment (CALDATA)," Report to the State of California Department of Alcohol and Drug Programs by National Opinion Research Center and Lewin-VHI, Inc. (April 1994).

How Should Low-Level Drug Dealers Be Punished?

Jonathan P. Caulkins
Philip B. Heymann

About 1.5 million people are arrested in the United States for drug-related violations every year.[1] How should the ones who are convicted be punished? Most people agree that high-level drug dealers or "kingpins" should be locked away for a long time. Likewise there is a promising new approach for nonviolent drug users, alternately called coerced treatment or coerced abstinence and described in Chapter 6 of this book. But what should be done with the more than one million low-level dealers who move drugs from the kingpins to the consumers? That straightforward question turns out to be surprisingly difficult to answer. The goal of this chapter is to provide a framework for thinking about how such offenders should be sentenced.

By many measures this is a large problem. Of the 1.5 million people arrested for drug law violations each year, about 375,000 are arrested for drug distribution, and about half of them are convicted.[2] Ninety percent of those convicted at the federal level and 70 percent of those convicted at the state level are incarcerated (Maguire and Pastore 1998, 394, 423). About 100,000 are sent to prison, with an estimated average time served of 33 months (ibid., 431). At an average incarceration cost of $25,000 per prison-cell-year (Caulkins et al. 1997), that represents an investment of about $7 billion annually on imprisonment of drug dealers, with additional billions spent on enforcement, adjudication, and jail sentences. By way of comparison, total federal spending on drug treatment and prevention is about $2.5 billion and $1.4 billion, respectively (ONDCP 1997, 19); state and local spending on these programs is of a comparable magnitude (ONDCP 1993).

For two reasons low-level dealers absorb the vast majority of this enforcement effort. First, low-level dealers are easier to arrest because they operate in more public locations and participate in transactions which are of lower value, limiting the precautions that can practically be taken per transaction. Second, there are vastly more of them because drug dealers at one level of the distribution network sell to multiple individuals at the level below (Caulkins 1997). To illustrate, suppose there were five layers of dealers, with importers or manufacturers at the top and retail dealers at the bottom, and suppose that every dealer supplied eight people. Then there would be over 60 times as many retailers and first-level wholesale dealers as there would be dealers in the top three layers of the distribution network combined.

One could address sentencing decisions for each of these layers separately, but as a first pass we simply want to differentiate between sentencing for "high level" and "low level" dealers, with the presumption that high-level dealers should receive long sentences but that sentencing of lower-level dealers merits some analysis. We could define everybody above retail to be "high level," but that is problematic for conceptual and practical reasons. Conceptually, first-level wholesale dealers are very far from "kingpins" in terms of wealth, power, and amounts of drugs sold. Pragmatically, it is not always easy for the criminal justice system to distinguish retail sellers from the lowest level of wholesale dealers. Hence we lump retail and first-level wholesale dealers together and discuss sentencing of "low-level" rather than just "retail" dealers. Moreover, there is a great deal of cycling between these two levels.

There is enormous heterogeneity in the sanctions these low-level drug dealers receive. About a quarter of those convicted of drug trafficking are sentenced to nothing more than probation (ibid., 427).[3] Yet some receive non-parolable life terms, and in California there are circumstances under which even a misdemeanor drug conviction must be given a minimum sentence of 25 years to life.[4] These sharp contrasts in sentencing show up between people possessing more or less than the threshold quantities that trigger mandatory minimum sentences, between people possessing powder vs. crack cocaine under the federal mandatory minimum system, and between states that have unusually tough sentencing laws, such as Michigan, and their neighbors, such as Wisconsin, that do not.

Much heterogeneity in sanctions is appropriate because there is a great deal of heterogeneity in the behavior of drug dealers. For example, not all dealers are equally violent. There are about 7,500 drug-related murders in the United States each year (Caulkins et al. 1997, 175–179), even though at least 1.5 million people have sold an illicit drug at the retail level in the past 12 months.[5] Thus in any given year at most one in every 200 drug dealers resorts to homicidal violence. Similarly, some but not all dealers employ juvenile runners or sell in front of treatment clinics. Some sell only marijuana; others sell heroin and crack. Some dealers are first-time adolescent offenders with no prior record; others are adult, repeat offenders with violent priors.

Unfortunately, the variability in sentences is not well correlated with the variability in culpability. This mismatch violates the fundamental tenet of justice that the punishment should fit the crime. It also represents a missed opportunity to intervene in drug markets in ways that reduce the damage drug dealers impose on society.

Developing more coherent and more effective policies is not an easy matter. Punishing purveyors of black-market products is tricky, and conventional models, whether conceptual or mathematical, do not apply. When we lock up a pathological rapist we lock up the rapes, reducing the rate at which the general citizenry is victimized. When we lock up a black-market distributor, of drugs or any other commodity, we create a job opening for someone else, and, to a considerable degree, those job openings are filled by replacement dealers (Kleiman 1997).

However, incarcerating dealers is believed to affect the amount of drugs sold to some extent. It makes drug dealing riskier, for which dealers presumably demand greater compensation. To the extent that they do, this raises the price of drugs and, hence, reduces consumption (Reuter and Kleiman 1986). Enforcement can make dealers more cautious, which should make transactions more difficult to complete (Moore 1973). Finally, if the incarceration is focused on dealers who are unusually noxious and their replacements are merely average, then enforcement may help reduce the violence, disorder, and other negative externalities associated with drug markets (Caulkins 1992). However, it is not the case that incarceration incapacitates drug dealing the way it does non-consensual crime.

Hence, to address the important question of how low-level drug dealers should be punished, it is important to start with a clean slate. At some basic level, there are two motivations for punishing criminals. We punish criminals simply because we think it is the just or moral thing to do, and we punish criminals in order to achieve tangible objectives, such as reducing crime. In the next two sections we take up the perspectives of justice and efficiency in turn. Drawing on insights developed in those sections, we then suggest ways in which sentencing policy toward low-level drug dealers might usefully be reformed.

What Is the Just Punishment for Low-Level Drug Dealing?

Issues of justice can be extraordinarily complicated. We wish to focus just on the notion that the "punishment should fit the crime," and within that paradigm we address just two issues. First, is the average level of punishment appropriate? Second, are longer (shorter) than average sanctions being directed at those dealers who are above (below) average in terms of the threat they pose to society?

How Tough Are We on Drug Dealers Generally?

Whether the average sanction imposed on low-level drug dealers is too severe, about right, or not severe enough is a matter for personal values and opinion, but it is useful to compare sanctions for drug selling with those imposed for other crimes. Relatively speaking, are we tough on drug dealers? The answer depends on how one measures severity.

The minimum time served for a federal conviction for distributing 50 grams of crack cocaine (less than one-millionth of annual United States consumption) is 10 years, which is also about the average time served for murder or non-negligent manslaughter.[6] In New York State both murder and selling two ounces of cocaine are class A-I felonies; both rape and selling one vial of crack are class B felonies (Paul Schectman, personal communication). However, the actual time served may be reduced by plea bargaining and, in states that do not have truth-in-sentencing laws, prison "release valves."[7] For example, in New York someone charged with selling two ounces of cocaine could be prosecuted for an A-I felony, with a minimum sentence of 15 years to life. More likely, he or she would plead to a lesser charge. Even if the charge were reduced just one step to an A-II felony, the sentence would be three years to life. With a three-year lower end of the sentence range, the individual becomes eligible for a six-month shock ("boot camp") program. Those who complete the program are eligible for parole, and 90 percent are released immediately. So a minimum sentence of 15 years to life often results, in practice, in less than a year served.[8]

In part because of plea bargaining and these "release valves" and in part because of the enormous number of drug sales, the expected incarceration time for making a drug sale is only about an hour. This is two orders of magnitude less than the expected incarceration time for a burglary, robbery, or car theft.[9]

Some would justify or criticize our present sentences in terms of the number of violent or property crimes drug offenders commit. If a typical retail cocaine seller committed all of the non-consensual crimes associated with both the distribution and consumption of the cocaine he or she sold in a year, the expected incarceration time would be one to one and a half months (Caulkins 1996). That is about half the time he or she should expect to serve for selling that cocaine.[10]

The expert consensus is that the United States today is highly punitive toward drug sellers when compared to other Western industrialized countries (MacCoun and Reuter 1998) or to ourselves 15 years ago (Reuter 1992, 1997). Indeed, the strictness of the Rockefeller Drug Laws in New York State was the subject of a recent Human Rights Watch Report (Human Rights Watch 1997).

The American public, in contrast, does not seem to think that low-level drug dealers are punished too severely. Survey respondents from the general population prefer punishments for low-level dealers greater than those specified in the federal sentencing guidelines. Similarly, a 1995 Gallup poll found that 84 percent of the public favored increasing criminal penalties for drug offenders, and only 14 percent thought law enforcement was doing enough to convict and punish people for the use and sale of illegal drugs (Maguire and Pastore 1996, 168).

There are at least three interpretations of this discordance between the wishes of the people and the judgment of the experts. The values of the experts may be systematically more liberal and more lenient than those of the masses.[11] Or experts may understand things about drug dealing that are relevant to its punishment and that are not widely appreciated. For instance, laypeople may not realize how many dealers there are and, hence, may believe each dealer is responsible for a greater portion of the drug problem than is in fact the case. Likewise, laypeople may not appreciate the extent to which incapacitation for consensual crimes such as drug dealing is undermined by replacement. Or the public may be more distressed by aspects of the punishment process, such as pretrial release, than by sentence length, but express that frustration through calls for tougher sanctions.

Are We Tough on the Right Dealers?

Whatever the conclusion about whether we are sufficiently tough on low-level drug dealers on average, one might also be interested in how well correlated the heterogeneity in punishment is with heterogeneity in culpability within the class of low-level drug dealers. The short answer is deficiently and perhaps not well at all.

Often sentences are governed primarily by the amount of drug possessed, but amount possessed can be a poor indicator of the importance of the defendant (Caulkins et al. 1997). High-level dealers generally hire others, sometimes called "couriers" or "mules," to physically possess the drugs the dealer owns and controls. In those cases, the risks associated with possession, including the risks of long sentences, fall on mere employees of the drug-distribution system, not on those who own or control the drugs. Weight-driven sentences also create sharp differences in sentence length based on small differences in weight (just below vs. just above a threshold trigger quantity), location (for example, in Michigan vs. Wisconsin), or type of drug (powder vs. crack cocaine).

Furthermore, sentences are typically based on the total weight of any mixture containing a detectable quantity of a controlled substance, not on the amount of the drug itself. Thus, possessing 8 grams of pure cocaine is punished less severely than possessing 10 grams of a powder that is only 10 percent cocaine by weight.

Other reasons why heterogeneity in time served is not well correlated with heterogeneity in culpability are less obvious. Most people charged with drug trafficking plead guilty, presumably to a lesser charge with a shorter sentence. The criminal justice system is spared an expensive trial; the defendant is spared the risk of a very long term. That means that the individuals who get the longest sentences are the ones who refused to accept a plea bargain; some of them are people whose roles were so peripheral that they mistakenly believed they would not be convicted in a trial (see Cohen 1997).

A similar perversity can occur with federal mandatory minimum sentences. The only way to avoid such a sentence is by offering "substantial assistance" to prosecutors in pursuit of other criminals. This occurs in about 15 percent of federal mandatory minimum cases (GAO 1993). In general, larger drug dealers have more information to offer prosecutors than mules or couriers do, so again the longest sentences may fall on some of the least culpable (Schulhofer 1989).

As mentioned above, prison systems have developed "release valves" to help relieve overcrowding. Unfortunately eligibility for a release valve may have next to nothing to do with how dangerous an offender is. For example, 32 percent of those who enter the New York State shock incarceration program fail to complete the program, typically because they cannot handle its structure and discipline. Those who fail must serve their minimum sentence. There is little reason to believe that vicious, professional dealers are more likely to fail and, hence, serve a longer term, than are drug abusers who support their habit through infrequent low-level selling.

Similarly, eligibility criteria for New York State's work release and Comprehensive Alcohol and Substance Abuse Treatment (CASAT) programs include having no prior history of absconding. Again, vicious but disciplined individuals may serve shorter sentences than others who are less dangerous but who have been less disciplined in the past. More generally, prison officials are motivated primarily by a desire to relieve overcrowding, not by a desire to ensure that the most culpable are held the longest. Even if prison administrators wanted to be selective in whom they released, they do not have ready access to as much information as is available to prosecutors and judges. Official criminal justice histories may give a less nuanced image of how dangerous an individual dealer is than could a community affairs officer from the neighborhood or a local prosecutor.

At one level the inability of the criminal justice system to ensure that the most dangerous dealers serve the longest sentences sparks a sense of outrage. At another, it is quite understandable. Time served is determined by decisions made by individuals in many agencies (district attorneys' offices, courts, the prison system, and so on), representing multiple levels of government (city, county, state) and multiple branches of government (police from the executive branch, judges from the judiciary, laws set by the legislature), who often have conflicting objectives (for example, the police may try to arrest as many people as possible and prison officials may strive to reduce overcrowding). The system evolved while processing people who committed violent and property crimes, but an increasing fraction of those in the system are there for the consensual crime of selling drugs. Official records are the primary means of transmitting information across agency and jurisdictional boundaries, but those records carry little of the information that can meaningfully differentiate the merely bad dealers from the truly awful. In some respects the criminal justice system resembles an old country house that has grown over time and, though functional, is awkward.

That the failure to match sanction severity to culpability is explicable does not imply that it should be tolerated. Important policy decisions and interventions are being made in a not particularly coherent manner. The nature of the problem makes clear, though, that it cannot be substantially ameliorated by tweaking rules at the margin. For example, the much-discussed proposal to shrink or eliminate the gap between crack and powder sentences under federal mandatory minimums might mollify those who view the disparity as discriminatory, but it would affect the sentencing of only a very small proportion of convicted low-level dealers. The problem is structural and can be summarized in three points.

- Determining sentences at the state (or federal) level with formulas based on a small set of consistently observable criteria (such as quantity possessed) results in "excessive uniformity" (Schulhofer 1989) and fails to assign the toughest sentences to the most blameworthy dealers because important case-specific information is overlooked.
- High minimum sentences imply that all but the most egregious offenders receive the minimum sentences. They also give prosecutors so much power to induce pleas that injustices can result.
- High case volumes make it difficult to examine cases on their individual merits. Coupled with high minimum sentences, they overwhelm the correctional system, leading to the development of release valves that substantially reduce time served for a subset of those sentenced, and there is little reason to think that the reductions are targeted at the least dangerous or the least culpable offenders.

This discussion of how "just" are the sentences for low-level dealers can be summarized as follows. Whether the average sanction is more or less severe than the sanction for comparable non-consensual crimes depends on how one measures severity and what crimes one thinks are comparable. Experts tend to think the average sanction is too high; the public thinks it is too low. What can be concluded more definitely is that the heterogeneity in sanction severity both within and between states is not well correlated with heterogeneity in culpability. Furthermore, the sources of the disparities stem from the basic structure of the system.

What Is the Effective Punishment for Low-Level Drug Dealing?

Ineffectiveness of "Muddling Through"

When it comes to punishing low-level drug dealers, the criminal justice system has been, to use Lindblom's term, "muddling through" (Lindblom 1959). As we have seen, that approach has not produced a *just* system of punishments, at least by our definition of what is just.

Past research has shown that it has also failed to produce a system that is *effective* at achieving tangible policy objectives. Our primary interest is not in revisiting these criticisms of effectiveness but in suggesting how the system might be improved, so we will only sketch the broad outlines of those arguments.

Since the early 1980s the United States has greatly increased the number of dealers incarcerated, both in absolute terms and relative to any growth in the market, but there is little evidence that this reduced drug use or drug-related crime. During the period when policy was becoming progressively tougher toward dealers, trends in drug use and drug-related violence were not monotonic. During the late 1980s drug-related violence grew, but drug use fell. In the 1990s violence fell, but use among youth rose while overall prevalence held relatively steady. So depending on the time period and the measure selected, one can find a positive or negative correlation between sentencing stringency and drug-related outcomes. Reviewing this evidence, Reuter (1997, 267) concludes that "increasing toughness has not accomplished its immediate objectives of raising price and reducing availability."

Similar conclusions are reached from other perspectives. Model-based studies of the cost-effectiveness of different interventions have concluded that expanding the sort of drug enforcement the United States now pursues would reduce drug use and drug-related crime, but it would achieve those benefits only at great cost (e.g., Rydell and Everingham 1994; Caulkins et al. 1997). Many factors contribute to this conclusion, including replacement of incarcerated dealers, markets' ability to displace and adapt, inability to target long sentences on the right dealers, and the high public cost of incarceration. These studies conclude that other interventions would be substantially more cost-effective at reducing both drug use and drug-related crime. Furthermore, for other types of crime, it appears that well-designed sentencing policies can reduce crime much more cost-effectively than can some current mandatory sentencing policies (Greenwood et al. 1994)

Given that the past approach of muddling through has created a system which does not seem to be either just or particularly effective, one might be tempted to try to approach the problem from a more comprehensive and rational framework.

Impracticality of a Top-down Rational Approach

To approach the problem of sentencing low-level drug dealers systematically, one must begin by acknowledging that there are multiple relevant goals, and that no single sentencing policy is best with respect to every goal. To illustrate, one goal might be to reduce drug use. Another could be minimizing the cost to the taxpayers of incarcerating drug dealers. Making sentences tougher might help with respect to the first goal but be counterproductive with respect to the second. As another example, the deterrence power of a fixed number of prison cells is greater if they are used to give a larger number of shorter sentences than if offenders are subject to a lower probability of getting a very long sentence. That is, certainty matters more than severity (Blumstein and Nagin 1977; Nagin 1998). However, there is evidence that any spell of incarceration, no matter how long, can reduce one's potential earnings in the legal job market (Freeman 1995). Thus giving many people short sentences might do more to reduce drug use, but it might also have a greater adverse impact on the number of dealers who can find productive work in legitimate enterprises.

Not only are there multiple, conflicting goals, but there also is no universal rule for weighting or combining them into one summary measure. Some people might care a great deal about reducing drug use. Others might care more about reducing drug-related crime. Still others might value most highly a reduction in our reliance on incarceration or the number of minority males who are disenfranchised by receiving a felony drug conviction.

Adding to the complexity, there are alternative enforcement policies, and the choices go beyond simply picking an average sentence severity. As a society we could arrest more or fewer drug dealers by expanding or contracting the intensity of drug law enforcement, or we could change the procedures for determining which dealers get the longest sentences.

To help order this complexity, one could create a matrix with a row for each sentencing alternative and a column for each outcome or goal. The entries of the matrix would indicate how effective each alternative is at achieving each goal. Table 8.1 shows an example of such a matrix.

Obviously one could refine Table 8.1 by adding more rows and/or columns. Likewise, one could imagine composite policies that combined the themes of two or more of the given rows. Furthermore, one would like to have more detailed descriptions of what the various rows and columns mean to ensure a common, unambiguous understanding. The matrix in Table 8.1 is meant to be illustrative, not definitive.

Theoretically, experts could fill in such a matrix with descriptions of the likely impact of each sentencing alternative on each outcome. Then every decisionmaker, whether a legislator, a voter, or a member of a sentencing commission, could draw inferences from the completed matrix. For example, if the decisionmaker cared most about one or a few goals (columns), he or she could support whatever sentencing option (row) was judged to be most effective at achieving those goal(s). Or, if one row were inferior to another row with respect to every attribute about which the decisionmaker cared, the decisionmaker could rule out the sentencing policy represented by the first row.

Unfortunately, using such a matrix is not likely to be a practical way to compute the optimal policy. Distressingly little is understood about how drug markets respond to sentencing changes, so there is enormous uncertainty concerning many if not most of the cells in the matrix, particularly those concerning how interventions would affect behavior outside the criminal justice system (such as levels of drug use and levels of drug-related crime) as opposed to inside (numbers of trials, people incarcerated, and so on).[12] There are methods for dealing with such uncertainty. As posed, the problem of choosing a sentencing strategy is a classic multi-attribute decision problem (Keeney and Raiffa 1976). However, the standard tools are unlikely to be useful in this context because there are too many decisionmakers. Applying the standard tools is an elaborate and time-consuming process. If there were just one or a few decisionmakers, it might be worth the investment. However, there are literally thousands of stakeholders, each with a diffuse interest, and it is not practicable for each to work through the exercise of identifying weights, quantifying uncertainty, eliciting utility functions, and so on.

Table 8.1 Illustrative matrix of sentencing options and outcomes

	Public outcomes					CJS effects			Justice
	Use by current users and related problems	Initiation of new users	Harm to dealers and their families	Drug-related crime and violence	Community effects (other than crime and violence)	Cost of enforcement /prison	Number of trials	Ability to prosecute higher-level dealers	Public sense of justice about system
B1 Status quo									
B2 Status quo w/half as many arrests									
B3 More certain but shorter sentences									
B4 More certain and more severe									
B5 Focus on recidivists									
B6 Focus on amount sold									
B7 Focus on context of dealing									

Descriptions of sentencing options:

B1: Status quo: A mixture of sentences from 0 (if the case is not prosecuted or the sentence is probation) to 5 years or more, depending largely on prior drug convictions and the amount of drugs possessed at the time of arrest. Currently, half those arrested are convicted. Of those, 27% receive a sentence of probation, 22% jail, and 51% prison.

B2: Status quo with half as many drug arrests: Cut enforcement in half by reducing all types of drug arrests by 50%. No change in the type of arrests made, the probability of conviction given arrest, the probability of conviction given prosecution, or the distribution of sanctions given conviction.

B3: More certain but shorter sentences: Increase by 50% the number of people incarcerated by increasing prosecution given arrest and reducing the probability of probation given conviction. Reduce length of longer sentences by enough to hold constant the number of people incarcerated.

B4: More certain and more severe sentences: Two-to-five-year sentences for everyone convicted of drug selling who does not offer substantial assistance in developing a case against someone else.

B5: Focus on recidivists: First-time offenders would receive probation, a suspended sentence, or a diversionary punishment that does not create a criminal record. Subsequent convictions would lead to sentences comparable to those given today, with longer sentences for those with the longest records.

B6: Focus on amount sold: Sentences would increase sharply with the amount possessed and/or the amount found to have been sold previously. E.g., sanctions for cocaine might be one week for a gram or less, two months for 1–10 grams, one year for 10–100 grams, five years for 100–1,000 grams, and more than five years for more than a kilogram.

B7: Focus on context of dealing: The base sentence for drug dealing would be no more than six months for low-level selling, but there would be significant (e.g., five-year) add-ons for selling while in possession of a firearm, employing a minor in the drug trade, exercising violence in the course of drug dealing, selling within a certain distance of a school or drug treatment clinic, open and notorious taking over of a neighborhood, etc.

A more fundamental problem, though, may be with the perspective Table 8.1 encourages one to adopt, both with respect to jurisdiction and with respect to scope within the criminal justice system. The questions raised by the table implicitly adopt a state-level perspective because they focus on formal sentencing policy, which is now made primarily by legislatures and sentencing commissions. However, any given policy could have different effects in different communities and at different stages in an epidemic of drug abuse. That is, the entries in the matrix may vary across communities and over time.

Furthermore, the table focuses attention on the question of how long a convicted dealer should be incarcerated, but that decision is just one of a set of policies that collectively determine which dealers will be punished and how. Policies of the police, prosecutors, prisons, probation, and parole also matter.

These observations might be summarized as follows. It is common to address the question of what should be done with low-level drug dealers by thinking broadly in jurisdictional terms (state-level policies) but narrowly within the overall flow of criminal justice system processing (focusing on sentence given conviction). Perhaps just the opposite perspective would be more appropriate, thinking in terms of smaller jurisdictions but encompassing arrest, prosecution, and the adjudication and punishment processes more generally, not just sentencing.

We will explore this proposition in two ways. First, we will elaborate on some of the disadvantages of the "state level, sentence given conviction" perspective relative to a "local level, entire punishment process" perspective. Then we will propose a mechanism for shifting decisionmaking over sentencing from the state level to a more local level. Some might argue that the greatest potential for improving the current system is associated not with the shift from "state" to "local level" but with moving from the "sentence given conviction" to the "entire punishment process" perspective. Indeed, we will briefly mention a few such opportunities.

Given the earlier discussion of heterogeneity in the destructiveness of dealing behaviors, the analysis below will assume that an ability to selectively target sanctions is desirable. Giving tougher sanctions to the worst offenders is not only just but also pragmatic; through both incapacitation and deterrence, it has the capacity to push dealing into less destructive forms even when it cannot suppress dealing alto-gether.[13] In particular, we have in mind that some small fraction (per-haps 5–10 percent) of low-level dealers stand out from the rest as un-usually vicious or destructive and that on both justice and efficiency grounds it would be desirable to target those dealers with unusually long prison terms. By definition, selectivity implies that the other low-level drug dealers would be treated more leniently. This philosophy has something in common with the 1980s priority-prosecution pro-gram for special violent offenders (Moore et al. 1984) and is appeal-ing in view of indications that recent successes in crime control stem from the use of community policing and community prosecution to target the most dangerous individuals.

Some might wonder whether local agencies know who the most dangerous offenders are, but acquiring such knowledge is a central objective of community policing and recent interventions show it is eminently feasible. For example, the Boston Gun Project (Kennedy 1997) demonstrated that the identities of the most violent offenders were known to the police so well that the project team could meet with them and their gangs. The characteristics that make such individ-uals a great concern, such as their repeat serious offending, also make them vulnerable to criminal justice intervention. Kennedy (1997, 461) describes the "enormous sanctioning power that the enforcement community could bring to bear against particular gangs and gang members" through cooperation of a collection of agencies including local police, federal agencies, parole, probation, youth outreach work-ers, school police, and others. Conspicuously absent from Kennedy's list is formal sentencing, which is seen as relatively unhelpful in its present form. Our proposal is intended to help make sentencing re-sponsive to how dangerous the community perceives offenders to be so that it can play a greater role in responding to the concentration of serious offending among a minority of all offenders.

Problems with a "State Level, Sentence Given Conviction" Perspective

In theory state-level sentencing policy can focus severe sanctions on the most destructive dealers by giving short sentences for dealing itself and augmenting those sentences with significant legislated add-ons for particularly destructive forms of dealing. However, the results of past efforts to write such a focus into sentencing policy have been discouraging. For example, in Massachusetts the School Zone Statute imposes a mandatory two-year sentence on those caught dealing within 1,000 feet of a school (Massachusetts General Laws, C.94C, s.32J). That sounds like a useful distinction until one realizes that most parts of most urban areas are within 1,000 feet of a school, so the statute does not achieve much in the way of focusing. In New York State, a similar statute raises the felony level by one for selling to someone under the age of 18 near a school. However, minors who buy drugs are not likely to turn in their supplier, and if a police officer poses as a 16-year old, the charge in New York would be "attempted" sale to a minor near a school because the police officer is not actually under the age of 18. Attempted felonies are charged at one level below the level for completed offenses. So attempted sale to a minor near a school would be charged at the same level as a completed sale generally is. As a result, the New York State school zone statute has almost no effect on enforcement or sentencing (Paul Schectman, personal communication). Even add-ons for possessing a firearm while dealing may be less useful than it would at first seem since dealers often keep their guns in their apartments instead of on their persons. Inasmuch as the law is what deters dealers from carrying their guns, the law may be reducing the incidence of spontaneous lethal violence, but it has not succeeded in "disarming" dealers if they can go back to their apartments at any time and retrieve a gun.[14]

The need for, and difficulty of, identifying and targeting particular behaviors is complicated by the interaction between behaviors and contexts. A policy that is effective at targeting long sentences at the worst dealers in one community or at one time might not achieve the same result elsewhere. A rural area might be well-advised to protect its children by enhancing sanctions for selling drugs within 1,000 feet of a school, but the same statute could have absolutely no ability to target the worst dealers in an urban area where every streetcorner is within 1,000 feet of a school. The urban area may prefer to focus sanctions on dealers who operate within 500 feet of a school or perhaps discard a distance criterion altogether and focus instead on those who employ youth as runners or lookouts, regardless of the location.

One neighborhood may have particular problems with streetcorner markets and want to punish public dealing severely; the same policy could be perverse in a neighborhood where crack houses are associated with more violence than are street markets.

Likewise drug markets and market behaviors are constantly evolving, so the type of dealing that constitutes the gravest threat to a community may change over time. Ideally policy should be able to respond to these changes by quickly increasing and decreasing sanctions for particular behaviors as they become more or less problematic. Unfortunately, these changes can occur more often and more quickly than state legislatures can redesign sentencing statutes. Also, although legislatures have increased sanctions on certain behaviors as they have become problematic, they have not demonstrated a similar ability to reduce sanctions on behaviors as they become less problematic. This asymmetry tends to drive up average sentence length over time, thereby undermining efforts to selectively target the worst offenders.

Opportunities Suggested by a "Local Level, Entire Punishment Process" Perspective

This inability to achieve the desired focus through mandatory sentences triggered by statutory provisions can be contrasted with the large number of opportunities for useful reform suggested by a "local level, entire punishment process" perspective. In the next section we describe in detail a suggestion for how sentencing decisions might be moved to the local level, but first we briefly sketch possibilities arising at other stages of the punishment process.

Arrest. Police have considerable potential to focus punishment on particular subsets of dealers by focusing arrests on those groups. Arresting as many low-level dealers as possible is not the best strategy. Large numbers of arrests force the rest of the criminal justice system into mass production mode, making it harder to make distinctions among different types of dealers. If the police arrested fewer people but increased the proportion who were particularly vicious, that would go a long way toward achieving the desirable results even if the rest of the system continued to operate as before.

Prosecution.   Current tough sentencing laws give prosecutors considerable power to induce defendants to plead guilty to some lesser charge. That power is not typically used, however, to differentiate unusually vicious dealers from run-of-the-mill dealers. The crush of heavy caseloads encourages setting plea policies based on the simplest facts, such as "First-time offenders charged with a class B felony will be given the chance to plead to a class D felony." A superior strategy might be to invest more prosecutors' time on each case, talking with police about the defendant, examining past arrests to see if they were overcharged misdemeanors or reflected true felonious behavior, and so on. Then for the subset of charged dealers who seem to pose the gravest threat to the community, the prosecutor might offer only the chance to plead to a class C felony, not a class D.

This would increase case-processing time, require better information-retrieval systems, and increase the number of trials. Applying greater discretion would require greater resources, but the cost of those resources would be small compared to the potential benefit of improving the effectiveness of drug enforcement. The situation is similar to the bumper sticker slogan "If you think education is expensive, try ignorance." If doubling case-processing expenditures improved the efficiency of incarceration by even 10 percent, in the sense of being able to use 10 percent fewer prison cells to keep the same number of particularly vicious offenders behind bars, the same level of public safety could be achieved at less cost to the taxpayers.[15]

Pretrial release.   One source of public mistrust of the current system is the observation that drug dealers arrested today are often out selling on the street tomorrow. That can happen when arrest does not lead to incarceration. It can also happen if arrest leads to a very long prison sentence—if that sentence is imposed after a period of pretrial release. Judges can make pretrial release conditional on a variety of behaviors, not just posting bail. This discretion might be used more aggressively than it is currently. For example, it could be a routine condition of release that arrestees not enter the neighborhood where they were arrested or any other known dealing locations.

Community supervision. Another source of public frustration with current processing of convicted drug dealers is that those sentenced to probation can resume their dealing activities with relative impunity. Coerced abstinence (discussed in Chapter 6) responds to the observation that a large proportion of the cocaine and heroin used in the United States is consumed by people who are nominally under criminal justice supervision. In particular, it responds by using a technology (drug testing) to closely monitor behavior between contacts with criminal justice system personnel (such as probation officers). One could imagine a parallel approach to controlling drug dealing, and criminal activity more generally.

A distressing proportion of crimes—including drug dealing—are committed by people on probation or parole. Technology could be employed to monitor the behavior of these individuals between contacts with the criminal justice system. For example, those under supervision could be required to wear a transponder that would pinpoint their location at all times to within a few meters. This would facilitate verification of compliance with positive terms of release, such as attending drug treatment or maintaining employment, and enhance enforcement of prohibitions against entering known drug markets. The system could even include an alarm that would sound if the individual entered a proscribed area. If crimes were logged into a geographic information system, that system could list all probationers and parolees who were in the area of the crime during the period when the crime occurred.

Proposal for Shifting Sentencing to the Local Level

Adopting a "local level, entire punishment process" perspective presents many opportunities for reforms that would improve the punishment and control of low-level drug dealers. In the interests of brevity, we detail only one—shifting sentencing decisionmaking power away from state (and federal) institutions (legislatures, sentencing commissions, and prison authorities who implement release valves) to the criminal justice system operating at the local level. We stress the generality of the term "criminal justice system" in the latter option. We are not advocating a return to the old system of judicial discretion, but rather envision a partnership of judges, prosecutors, and police working together to solve the problem of identifying and targeting those low-level drug dealers who are the most destructive to their communities.

Such a shift is not without its disadvantages, so before we describe how such a system might work, it is important to consider what are desirable characteristics of a system for sentencing low-level offenders.

Desirable Characteristics of a Sentencing System

In addition to the capacity to identify and target behaviors that are particularly noxious in a given context, one would like a sentencing system to be manageable, to not violate norms of equity, to send a clear warning for purposes of deterrence, and to give those making sentencing decisions an incentive to consider the opportunity cost of giving out long sentences. We contrast the current approach with the alternative of control by local criminal justice systems with respect to these four characteristics.

Manageability. In order for a government entity to use policy to achieve ends the public desires, the government entity must be cognizant of and responsive to the public's desires, the policy must actually be implemented, and implementing the policy must have the expected desirable effects.

It is not clear whether moving sentencing decisions to the local level would make them more or less responsive to the public's desires. State legislators are elected, but so are most prosecutors and some judges. Other law enforcement officials are generally not elected, but neither are sentencing commissions, and both are fairly responsive to elected officials.

It seems probable, however, that policies devised by local criminal justice systems would be more likely to be implemented simply because local criminal justice systems play the dominant role in implementing sentencing policy. (Prison-release decisions would be the one aspect not directly under their control.) In contrast, it is not uncommon to hear of a state legislature's intentions being thwarted by the actions of local criminal justice systems. California judges ignoring prior convictions in order to avoid triggering a third-strike sentence of 25 years to life is a prime example.

Local control over sentencing policy may also offer a greater ability to predict the consequences of policy changes. It would certainly not be easy for a local criminal justice system to predict how drug use and selling in its community would respond to a policy change. But predicting statewide outcomes is even harder because it requires not only understanding effects at the community level but also achieving that understanding for many different communities and somehow "averaging" the different effects.

Equity.   Expanding local discretion raises concerns with accountability and potential abuse of power. State-level decisionmaking is not generally as vulnerable to abuses because policies are not made on a case-by-case basis, policies must be defended in public statements or documents, and departures from routine behavior, such as variations from presumptive guidelines, must be justified. Unless a system that involves local discretion has these three characteristics, as does the one we proposed, it may be inferior with respect to equity concerns.

Clear deterrent signal.   One might at first expect state-level decisionmaking to have the greatest potential to communicate a clear and credible threat to criminals, but plea bargaining and prison release valves can make the actual time served much less than the statute would predict, undermining the deterrent effect. Furthermore, criminals do not necessarily follow legislative actions closely, so street lore concerning sentencing policy is not always up to date or accurate.

Determining policy at the local level risks sending mixed messages because the policies are geographically fragmented. However, many low-level dealers operate within a relatively small geographic area, and local police can directly communicate the threat of tough sentences to offenders. For example, part of Boston's sharp decline in youth homicides has been attributed to police confronting gang leaders and threatening to come down hard on whichever gang was the first to break a truce.

Averting a tragedy of the commons.   Prison costs are borne by the entire state, not just a local community. This creates for community-level decisionmakers the potential for a tragedy of the commons, in which every community has an incentive to label all of its dealers as particularly dangerous and send them to prison at little cost to themselves but great cost to the rest of the state. To a significant degree this problem already exists even with sentences set at the state level, because charging decisions are made locally. Also, to the extent that a local community is reluctant to have its own people sent to prison for long periods of time, local control might moderate sentence length. Nevertheless, the problem of harmful local incentives to ignore costs that can be shifted to a common, shared cost-bearer could conceivably be even worse with local control.

An economist's answer might be to have each community pay for its share of prisoners in the state system. However, that could generate some of the same inequities between need and ability to pay that occur with public schools financed predominantly by property taxes. Indeed, Brownsberger and Piehl (1997) have shown just how concentrated the neighborhoods of incarcerated drug dealers are in urban poverty areas. An alternative would be to assign a "budget" limiting the number of people each community could have in prison for low-level drug dealing at any given time. That also might be too radical a change. A more mundane solution would have a periodic comparison of what proportion of dealers each prosecutor's office treats as particularly vicious with legislated targets concerning those proportions. Individual cases or criteria used to determine what constitutes a vicious case would remain purely local decisions.

Summary.   Giving local officials control would probably be superior to the current state-level approach with respect to ability to target long sentences on the most dangerous offenders and ability to adapt policy to spatial and temporal variation in the nature of the drug problem. It would offer some advantages with respect to being manageable and communicating a clear deterrent message. The biggest concerns pertain to equity and the possibility that every locality would have an incentive to label all of its offenders as deserving long sentences in (state-funded) prisons. However, the current system does quite badly on those dimensions already, so it is not clear that local control would be any worse.

A Proposed System

Since giving local criminal justice officials more control seems promising, it is worth asking: How would a sentencing structure that was respectful of these concerns operate? And to what extent would the values that have led the Congress and a number of states to create sentencing guidelines and even mandatory minimum sentences be sacrificed? A hard look suggests that we can design a system that preserves many of the benefits of recent sentencing changes without their enormous costs.

Guideline systems designed to limit judicial discretion and sentencing have four primary objectives. They are intended to prevent unfairness and bias in the different treatment by two judges of people who are morally and practically the same—that is, to prevent horizontal inequality. They are intended, through the elimination of parole that generally accompanies them, to obtain truth in sentencing—that is, an actual sentence which corresponds closely to the sentence announced by a judge. They are intended to guarantee that a high level of thought and information is brought to bear in deciding on a sentence. Finally, they are intended to guarantee that the precise punishment for a particular crime is made clear in the hope of maximizing the deterrence that comes with that punishment. When high mandatory minimums are imposed on the sentencing structure by the legislature, an additional purpose is obviously to convey the legislature's view of the seriousness of the offense.

The price of pursuing these purposes is inevitably a reduced capacity to recognize variations based on the differing life histories of different defendants. Disagreement about the moral significance of such factors makes the price less than it might seem. But another cost has been ignored. In reducing greatly the way sentences can vary with individual characteristics, the state and federal guidelines systems and the mandatory sentences have also reduced desirable variations of sentences which depend upon the differing situations two communities may face or the same community may face at two different times. And the structure of uniform sentences across a state prevents prosecutors and police from using the threat of more severe punishment to focus enforcement efforts strategically on particularly dangerous groups or individuals.

How can we respect most of the values that underlie the guideline systems without these costs? The answer is straightforward: we can design a system that gives judges greater discretion but simultaneously gives local prosecutors the ability to discourage judges from using that discretion to give lenient sentences to individuals who meet the local community's definition of unusually destructive dealers. The system would work like this.

The legislature or a sentencing commission in the state (or, for the federal system, in Washington) would define two ranges of allowable sentences. The tougher "A" range would apply, in jurisdictions where "community sentencing" was in effect, to individuals who met the community's definition of unusually destructive dealers. The "B" range, which would apply in all other cases, would be substantially broader than the range common in jurisdictions with determinant sentencing today. In particular, the lower end of the allowable range would be reduced; sanctions for typical dealers should be modest enough to preserve a sharp differential between sanctions for typical dealers and those for unusually destructive dealers.[16]

The "A" range would be narrower and would have a higher minimum sentence than the "B" range. The minimum sentence could be set aside where the defendant had provided needed information. Finally, the legislature or sentencing commission would specify an upper bound on the proportion of charged dealers one would expect to meet the criteria for "unusually destructive" dealing. This bound would help alleviate the tendency of local prosecutors to overuse expensive prison resources that are funded by state, not local, tax dollars.

The legislature or a sentencing commission would also specify the culpability factors which a smaller jurisdictional unit might consider relevant in defining aggravated dealing for purposes of the "A" range. The list of factors might be quite long, including the vulnerability of the customers sought, the danger of the drug, the amount of the drug, the violence or dangers of violence associated with the drug market, the likelihood that severe punishments in the particular location would reduce the availability of drugs, the effect on neighborhood life of the dealing, the impact on the neighborhood of drug sentences, and more. Then the legislature would announce that the narrower, more severe "A" sentencing range would apply only to defendants who met the criteria for being unusually destructive in any prosecutorial jurisdiction where "community sentencing" was in effect.

For these purposes, "community sentencing" would mean that the district attorney or his representatives had met with police and community groups from the neighborhoods or towns within his jurisdiction and discussed their views as to appropriate criteria for sentencing and that he had followed these meetings with a written policy statement as to the sentencing consequences he believed should be given to each of the culpability factors (a statement that would be readily available to voters).

Note that the district attorney would have a strong incentive to establish community sentencing; without it, he would not have a "stick" comparable to mandatory minimum sentences with which to induce cooperation. However, the fact that publicly announced criteria would have to be met for a dealer to be defined as unusually destructive would limit the prosecutor's ability to wield this heavy stick against defendants who played only a peripheral role in the drug-distribution system. This would ameliorate the problem of minor players who do not have useful information to offer being perceived as uncooperative and receiving very long sentences.

The local judge could set sentences anywhere within the broad "B" state-wide sentencing requirements in jurisdictions without community sentencing. Where community sentencing was in effect the narrower "A" ranges would be the presumptive guidelines for defendants who the prosecutor argues meet the local definition of unusually destructive dealers. The guidelines would be presumptive, allowing the judge to depart if he gave a written reason. (One valid reason would be that the prosecutor was trying to classify a larger proportion of defendants as unusually destructive than the legislature defined as being a reasonable upper bound.) However, public pressure would lead the judge to give very serious attention to the prosecutor's recommendation. Likewise, if the prosecutor's argument and judge's assent to that argument became part of the defendant's official record, that information could be available to prison officials deciding who should be eligible for early release programs.

The result of this system would be some, but limited, differences between two prosecutorial jurisdictions. It would also be different punishment schemes at different times within the same jurisdiction. But the basis would be stated in advance with a clarity that reduced substantially the chance of bias in individual cases by particular judges or prosecutors. The threat of punishment would be made clear for maximum deterrence but focused where the community wanted it. The public would understand the truth about the sentence being imposed. The sentence would be based on thought and information reflected in an explanation made public. The result might or might not be more severe sentences than those imposed at a state level. That would depend upon the views of the people in the jurisdiction about different types of drug dealing.

Summary and Recommendations

How to punish low-level drug dealers is an important policy issue, but the current system evolved in a haphazard manner into one that is neither particularly just nor particularly effective, in no small part because heterogeneity in punishment is not well correlated with heterogeneity in culpability. The remedy is not likely to be found in modifying state laws and guidelines mandating what sentences to give convicted defendants. Trying to systematically evaluate and compare state-level reforms is not practical because there are too many stakeholders, too many competing objectives, and too much uncertainty concerning the effects of possible policy changes. Furthermore, standard considerations (weight or type of drugs, prior record, and so on) do not adequately differentiate between typical and unusually vicious dealers, and that deficiency cannot be remedied by tinkering with drug statutes. Legislators attempting to write algorithms into statutory law that differentiate the worst dealers from the average dealers is a grievous example of bureaucratic micromanagement by people who are not experts. The true experts on what constitutes a particularly vicious dealer must reside at the local level because behaviors that are vicious in one community and time may not be as problematic in another.

Hence, we are more likely to find the remedy by looking beyond sentencing decisions (to include, for example, decisions about whom to arrest and prosecute and about how to control those not incarcerated) and by moving discretion over sentencing decisions to the local level. In other words, we advocate taking a "local-level, entire punishment process" perspective rather than a "state-level, sentence given conviction" perspective when trying to target the most severe sanctions on the most destructive forms of dealing.

We sketch some opportunities at the arrest, prosecution, pretrial release, and community supervision stages, but focus on a proposed system ("community sentencing") for achieving local control over sentencing decisions without reverting to the old system of pure judicial discretion. This system could be accomplished by implementing the following suggestions:

- Legislatures should allow local jurisdictions to apply tougher, tighter sentencing guidelines to the subset of dealers in their jurisdiction who meet that jurisdiction's definition of "unusually destructive" patterns of dealing. To do this they would (1) specify factors that a smaller jurisdiction could consider in designing community sentencing policies, (2) specify what the narrower ("A") guidelines are, and (3) specify an upper bound on the proportion of individuals who might be expected to be "unusually destructive."
- Legislatures should make the primary or default policy ("B" policy) be indeterminate sentencing for low-level dealers with ranges broad enough to permit departures either above or below the modal sentence.
- Prosecutors wishing to pursue a community sentencing model should consult with police and other local representatives and produce a written policy statement describing how factors from the specified list would affect prosecution decisions.
- Prosecutors should argue for tougher sentences for those individuals who meet the local definition of "unusually destructive" dealers up to the proportion set by the state legislature.

- Judges should sentence under the tougher "A" guidelines when prosecutors ask them to do so as long as the proportion of such requests is within the bound set by the legislature.

Notes

This chapter benefited from many ideas and insights contributed by members of the Harvard Mind/Brain/Behavior Interfaculty Initiative working group on drugs and addictions.

1. In 1996 there were an estimated 1,506,200 arrests for drug-related violations (Maguire and Pastore 1998, 324).
2. In 1996 an estimated 25 percent of the 1,506,200 arrests for drug abuse violations were for sale or manufacture (ibid., 363). In 1994, 16,197 people were convicted of drug trafficking in U.S. District Courts and 165,430 in State Courts, for a total of 181,627 convictions, relative to an estimated 365,000 arrests for sale or manufacture (27 percent of the then 1,351,200 arrests for drug abuse violations) (Maguire and Pastore 1996, 432; 1998, 421)
3. In Massachusetts, a Continuance Without Finding (CWOF) is a common disposition for first-time low-level drug dealers in some urban areas (Will Brownsberger, personal communication). In New York the most common dealing charge is a class B felony, which is pled to a class D felony, which is probation-eligible for first-time felons (Paul Schectman, personal communication).
4. Michigan has over 200 individuals serving non-parolable life terms for possessing 650 grams or more of cocaine or heroin. For 86 percent of them, this is their first prison sentence (Michigan Department of Corrections 1996). Under California's "Three Strikes and You're Out" law, a felony conviction for someone previously convicted of two serious crimes generates a sentence of 25 years to life. Under a separate statute, misdemeanor convictions are "promoted" to felonies for individuals on parole (Greenwood et al. 1994).
5. The retail value of the cocaine market was between $30 billion and $40 billion in the years 1988–1993 (ONDCP 1996). Reuter et al. (1990) estimate that a regular (more than once a week) cocaine retailer in Washington sold an average of $4,570 worth of cocaine a month (median was less than $3,600), and that there were 22 dealers for every 14 full-time-equivalent dealers. Thus, there are about $(22 \div 14) \times \$35B \div (\$4,570 \times 12$ months/yr.) = 1,003,000 retail cocaine dealers. The retail value of all illicit drugs sold in the United States is about $50 billion, so even if street

sellers of other drugs sold as much in dollar terms as do cocaine sellers, which is doubtful, there would still be at least ($50 billion ÷ $30 billion) × 1,003,000 = 1,433,000 retail sellers.

6. U.S. annual cocaine consumption is estimated to be 291 metric tons (Everingham and Rydell 1994), a substantial portion of which is consumed as crack. Maguire and Pastore (1998, 431) report that the average estimated time served for murder/manslaughter excluding negligent manslaughter is 126 months.

7. Indeed, less than 1 percent of those in New York Department of Corrections institutions in 1996 (695 of 69,709) were there for class A-I drug felonies (Paul Schectman, personal communication).

8. The average stay in the New York prison system for those who go through the shock incarceration program is 222 days, which is the six-month program plus about six weeks to get to the program through intake. All information on the shock diversion program is from Paul Schectman.

9. Retail drug sales total about $50 billion. If the average value of a retail sale is $20, that implies about 2.5 billion drug sales a year at the retail level alone. There are about 300,000 people incarcerated for drug selling at any given time, and there are $365.25 \times 24 = 8,766$ hours in a year, so there are about 2.63 billion hours of incarceration served for drug selling each year. Wilson and Abrahamse (1992, 377) estimate time served per offense to be 81 hours for burglary, 106 hours for auto theft, and 96 hours for robbery.

10. Reuter, MacCoun, and Murphy (1990, 96) estimate that a retail cocaine dealer in Washington, D.C., in 1987 could "expect to serve 2¼ months of prison time as a consequence of a year's selling." Nationally, if there are 1,000,000 active and 250,000 incarcerated retail cocaine sellers at any one time, then every year of selling leads, on average, to one-fifth of a year, or 2.4 months, incarcerated.

11. This interpretation is supported by the observation that there is similar disagreement between experts and the public with regard to penal policy generally, not just with respect to drug law violations (Wilson 1995).

12. The disagreement highlights the need for more research on how drug enforcement affects drug markets. As Reuter has observed (1997), the United States spends hundreds of millions of dollars trying to evaluate and improve the effectiveness of the few billion dollars it spends on drug treatment and prevention, but only a few million dollars studying or evaluating the much greater resources committed to enforcement and incarceration.

13. This parallels the ability of interdiction to push smugglers from one route or mode of shipment to another even though it cannot "seal the borders" (Caulkins, Crawford, and Reuter 1993).

14. Preventing dealers from carrying guns may also increase their vulnerability to robbery, and both retribution for past robberies and preemptive acts of violence by dealers to establish a reputation that deters robbery may be among the more common types of violence for dealers.
15. ONDCP (1993) reports that in 1991 drug-control spending by state and local governments for corrections was $6.827 billion, more than 10 times the $649 million that was spent on prosecution and legal services related to drug control.
16. As Bentham (1843) observed, "The great inconvenience resulting from the infliction of great punishment for small offenses, is, that the power of increasing them in proportion to the magnitude of the offense is thereby lost."

References

Bentham, Jeremy. 1843. "Principles of Penal Law." In *Jeremy Bentham's Works,* ed. J. Bowring, pt. 2, bk. 1, 399–402.

Blumstein, Alfred, and Daniel Nagin. 1977. "The Deterrent Effect of Legal Sanctions on Draft Evasion." *Stanford Law Review* 29, no. 2.

Brownsberger, William N., and Anne M. Piehl. 1997. "Profile of Anti-Drug Law Enforcement in Urban Poverty Areas in Massachusetts." Report submitted to the Robert Wood Johnson Foundation Substance Abuse Policy Research Program.

Caulkins, Jonathan P. 1992. "Thinking about Displacement in Drug Markets: Why Observing Change of Venue Isn't Enough." *Journal of Drug Issues* 22, no.1, 17–30.

———. 1996. "Are Drug Users Accomplices to Murder?" Manuscript.

———. 1997. "Modeling the Domestic Distribution Network for Illicit Drugs." *Management Science* 43, no. 10, 1364–71.

Caulkins, Jonathan P., Gordon Crawford, and Peter Reuter. 1993. "Simulation of Adaptive Response: A Model of Drug Interdiction." *Mathematical and Computer Modeling* 17, no. 2, 37–52.

Caulkins, Jonathan P., C. Peter Rydell, William L. Schwabe, and James Chiesa. 1997. *Mandatory Minimum Sentences: Throwing Away the Key or the Taxpayers' Money?* MR-827-DPRC. Santa Monica: Rand.

Cohen, Sharon. 1997. "One Short Ride Turns into a Lifetime for a Woman in Michigan Prison." *Los Angeles Times,* Sept. 7, A35–36.

Everingham, Susan S., and C. Peter Rydell. 1994. "Modeling the Demand for Cocaine." MR-332-ONDCP/A/DPRC. Santa Monica: Rand.

Freeman, Richard B. 1995. "The Labor Market." In James Q. Wilson and Joan Petersilia, eds., *Crime* (San Francisco: ICS Press), 171–192.

General Accounting Office (GAO). 1993. "Mandatory Minimum Sentences: Are They Being Imposed and Who Is Receiving Them?" GAO/GGD-94–13. Nov.

Greenwood, Peter W., C. Peter Rydell, Allan F. Abrahamse, Jonathan P. Caulkins, James Chiesa, Karyn E. Model, and Stephen P. Klein. 1994. "Three Strikes and You're Out: Estimated Benefits and Costs of California's New Mandatory Sentencing Law." MR-509-RC. Santa Monica: Rand.

Human Rights Watch. 1997. "Cruel and Usual: Disproportionate Sentences for New York Drug Offenders." *Human Rights Watch* 9, no. 2(B).

Keeney, Ralph L., and Howard Raiffa. 1976. *Decisions with Multiple Objectives: Preferences and Value Tradeoffs*. New York: John Wiley.

Kennedy, David M. 1997. "Pulling Levers: Chronic Offenders, High-Crime Settings, and a Theory of Prevention." *Valparaiso University Law Review* 31, no. 2, 449–484.

Kleiman, Mark A. R. 1997. "The Problem of Replacement and the Logic of Drug Law Enforcement." *Drug Policy Analysis Bulletin*, no. 3.

Langan, Patrick A., and Jodi M. Brown. 1997. "Felony Sentences in the United States, 1994." Bureau of Justice Statistics Bulletin NCJ-165149. Washington: U.S. Department of Justice.

Lindblom, Charles E. 1959. "The Science of 'Muddling Through'." *Public Administration Review* 19, no. 2, 79–88.

MacCoun, Robert J., and Peter Reuter. 1997. "Interpreting Dutch Cannabis Policy: Reasoning by Analogy in the Legalization Debate," *Science* 278, 47–52.

———. 1998. "Drug Control." In *Oxford Handbook on Crime Control* (Oxford: Oxford University Press), 207–238.

Maguire, Kathleen, and Ann L. Pastore, eds. 1996. *Sourcebook of Criminal Justice Statistics 1995*. U.S. Bureau of Justice Statistics. Washington: Government Printing Office.

———. 1998. *Sourcebook of Criminal Justice Statistics 1997*. U.S. Bureau of Justice Statistics. Washington: Government Printing Office.

Michigan Department of Corrections. 1996. "Prisoners Sentenced to Life Terms for Drug Law Offenses." Fact sheet, Nov. 15.

Moore, Mark H. 1973. "Policies to Achieve Discrimination in the Effective Price of Heroin." *American Economic Review* 63, 270–279.

Moore, Mark H., Susan R. Estrich, Daniel McGillis, and William Spelman. 1984. *Dangerous Offenders: The Elusive Target of Justice*. Cambridge, Mass.: Harvard University Press.

Nagin, Daniel. 1998. "Criminal Deterrence Research: A Review of the Evidence and a Research Agenda for the Outset of the 21st Century." In Michael Tonry, ed., *Crime and Justice: An Annual Review of Research*, vol. 23 (Chicago: University of Chicago Press), 1–42.

Office of National Drug Control Policy (ONDCP). 1993. "State and Local Spending on Drug Control Activities: Report from the National Survey of State and Local Governments." White Paper. Washington.

———. 1996. *The National Drug Control Strategy, 1996.* Washington: The White House.

———. 1997. *The National Drug Control Strategy, 1997.* Washington: The White House.

Reuter, Peter. 1992. "Hawks Ascendant: The Punitive Trend of American Drug Policy." *Daedalus* 121, no. 3, 15–52.

———. 1997. "Why Can't We Make Prohibition Work Better? Some Consequences of Ignoring the Unattractive." *Proceedings of the American Philosophical Society* 141, no. 3, 262–275.

Reuter, Peter, and Mark A. R. Kleiman. 1986. "Risks and Prices: An Economic Analysis of Drug Enforcement." In M. Tonry and N. Morris, eds., *Crime and Justice: An Annual Review of Research,* vol. 7 (Chicago: University of Chicago Press), 289–340.

Reuter, Peter, Robert MacCoun, and Patrick Murphy. 1990. *Money from Crime: A Study of the Economics of Drug Dealing in Washington, D.C.* R-3894-RF. Santa Monica: Rand.

Rhodes, William, Paul Scheiman, Tanutda Pittayathikhun, Laura Collins, and Vered Tsarfaty. 1995. *What America's Users Spend on Illegal Drugs, 1988–1993.* Washington: Office of National Drug Control Policy.

Rydell, C. P., and S. S. Everingham. 1994. "Controlling Cocaine: Supply versus Demand Programs." Santa Monica: Rand.

Schulhofer, Stephen J. 1989. "The Development of the Federal Sentencing Guideline for Drug Trafficking Offenses." *Criminal Law Bulletin,* 50–59.

Wilson, James Q. 1995. "Crime and Public Policy," In James Q. Wilson and Joan Petersilia, eds., *Crime* (San Francisco: ICS Press), 489–507.

Wilson, James Q., and Allan Abrahamse. 1992. "Does Crime Pay?" *Justice Quarterly* 9, no. 3, 359–377.

Reflections on Drug Policy and Social Policy | 9

David Boyum
Peter Reuter

Apart from the perennial but politically inconsequential legalization debate, most public discussion about policy toward the currently illicit drugs can be summarized in a handful of words: drug enforcement versus drug treatment.[1] Indeed, the history of American drug policy can largely be seen as a long-standing argument over whether drug abuse is best dealt with as a criminal or a medical problem.[2]

Note that in this conventional cops-versus-docs framing, drug policy does not stand on its own, but rather is linked to, or even subsumed under, two other areas of public policy: criminal justice and health care. That is understandable. Our current policy of drug prohibition defines drug selling and most drug use as criminal. Beyond that, the association of drug abuse and criminal activity is undeniable—in the largest U.S. cities, roughly four out of five arrestees test positive for illegal drugs when given urine tests.[3] And although the precise causal relationship between drugs and crime is complex and unsettled, it is widely recognized that suppressing certain drug markets and some kinds of use is central to crime control.[4]

Connections between drug abuse and health care are also plain. Drug abuse is a risk factor for a variety of acute and chronic health problems.[5] Much addiction is thought to be linked to genetic predispositions, and notwithstanding the reservations of some contributors to this book, addiction is increasingly defined as a disease. Addiction therapy is generally considered medical treatment, even though doctors often play a marginal role.[6] And many widely abused "illegal" drugs, such as cocaine and PCP, are in fact tightly regulated pharmaceuticals that are legally employed by physicians and veterinarians.

In short, there are obvious reasons why, in both academic analyses and government policy, drug policy is closely tied to criminal justice and health policy. But there are comparably important ties between drug abuse and problems that are the principal concern of social policy—problems such as poverty, family breakdown, inner-city deterioration, chronic unemployment, public housing, disability, and child abuse. Social policy may be able to substantially reduce drug problems, and drug policy can substantially affect social problems. Yet little attention is given to the potential connections between drug policy and social policy by either academics or policymakers.

In this chapter we explore the potential for improving drug policy and social policy by better coordinating their objectives and operations. We begin with a conceptual look at connections between drug and social policy, discussing why we might want to forge tighter links between the two. We then move to more practical considerations: the structure of current drug policy; the experience of a particular issue where efforts have been made to connect drug and social policy (the provision of public assistance to those with drug problems); and general political considerations of trying to bring together drug policy and social policy. We find that the prospects for such coordination are brighter in theory than in practice. One barrier is that the strategy formulation and program budgeting of current drug policy are circumscribed by the standard view of drug policy as supply reduction and demand reduction, thus excluding programs that lower adverse consequences indirectly, as many social programs might. Another barrier lies in the fact that the institutions of social policy are not designed—normatively, politically, or operationally—to deal with the problem of addiction. In light of these and other complicating political factors, we reach the conclusion that only modest steps toward linking drug policy and social policy are advisable.

The Case for Linking Drug and Social Policy

Drug abuse appears not only to increase the chance that individuals will engage in crime but also to raise the likelihood of behavior and conditions that are the object of social policy. It is very hard to estimate the marginal effect of drug abuse on problems such as homelessness, child abuse, poverty, and unemployment, but the high relative prevalence of drug abuse among populations with these problems cannot be fully explained by the fact that disadvantage makes drug abuse more likely.

As to prevalence, most studies suggest that at least one-third of the homeless have substance abuse problems, including both drugs and alcohol. The General Accounting Office estimates that the majority of foster care cases involve parental substance abuse, much of it related to illicit drugs. Other research indicates that, even after controlling for social, demographic, and psychiatric variables, substance abusers are over three times as likely to physically abuse their children.[7] Estimates of drug abuse among welfare recipients vary widely, but at a minimum, in the early 1990s dependence on illicit drugs appeared several times more common among welfare recipients than among the general population.[8]

These numbers suggest that reductions in drug abuse among at-risk groups could materially reduce certain social problems. Some targeted drug policy efforts might even be more effective at achieving social policy goals than some social policy interventions explicitly striving for those goals, or at least might make a substantial contribution. For example, it is possible that effective drug treatment could do more to help chronically unemployed drug abusers return to work than standard job training programs.

However, the causal link between drug use and social problems is not unidirectional; almost all of the social problems that we have mentioned contribute to drug abuse. There is credible, though not overwhelming, evidence that the failure of public housing projects to provide safe and supportive communities, the decreasing prevalence of two-parent families, the high levels of long-term unemployment in many urban communities, and so on, all exacerbate drug problems, whether by increasing use of illicit drugs, the involvement of young persons in selling those drugs, or the difficulty of desisting from regular drug consumption. Thus improvements in housing for the poor, more effective job training, better family-preservation services, and the like, might reduce the extent of drug abuse and/or ameliorate the harms from it. Drug policymakers might seek to influence these other areas of policymaking that are not normally taken to be directed to drug control.[9] This indeed is the standard liberal critique of drug policy even as a concept. In this view drug use and drug problems are simply the manifestation of deeper social problems, and policy should be directed at "root causes."[10]

In fact, in some instances, policies or programs with no explicit drug-control objectives turn out to have substantial impacts on drug problems, perhaps because they are so comprehensive. The Gatreaux program, which promoted the dispersion of poorer families into the suburbs of Chicago, has shown in moderately rigorous analyses substantial reductions in the criminal involvement of the children of the families that moved, when compared to a control group that mostly stayed in the old neighborhoods.[11] Though the drug use outcome was not reported for this population, it would be surprising if it were not much lower than in the control group.

Finally, almost any medical intervention offers an opportunity for detection and perhaps treatment of drug abuse problems. Programs that provide prenatal care to poor women increase the likelihood of detection of maternal substance abuse and may help persuade the mother to abstain or reduce consumption during the remainder of pregnancy, thus lowering the likelihood of a drug-damaged infant. The ophthalmologist testing a patient's eyesight or the pediatrician administering a general checkup to an adolescent is well situated to identify signals of current drug use. The doctor may also be a credible purveyor of a health-oriented message designed to reduce drug involvement.

All these are instances of individualized programs in which reduced drug use is an unintended but predictable consequence of a program with other objectives. Perhaps even more could be gained by making formal operational linkages between drug policy and social policy programs. A theme of several chapters in this book is that drug use is responsive to incentives and coercive interventions and that policy should take advantage of opportunities to apply such leverage. For example, central to the logic of the coerced abstinence programs that Mark Kleiman and William Brownsberger advance is the opportunity the criminal justice system has to identify, treat, monitor, and sanction the drug use of probationers and parolees. As we discuss below, many social welfare programs could in principle operate as similar mechanisms.

So far, we have reported only good news, where the main goal of drug policy (to reduce drug use) supports the goals of social policy (to alleviate social problems) and vice-versa. But there are also potential areas of conflict. Certain social policy programs may have an exacerbating effect on drug abuse. For example, public assistance, especially when given in cash or easily marketable vouchers such as food stamps, can provide resources for drug purchases. Even when given in the form of housing or medical insurance, both of which are relatively unmarketable, assistance may still free up for drug use money that would otherwise have been spent on housing or medical care.

By the same token, aspects of drug policy may be counterproductive from the perspective of certain social policy objectives. For instance, illicit drug markets spawned by prohibition appear to divert some inner-city adolescents and young adults from education and licit employment, in part because sentencing and other law enforcement policies advantage juveniles relative to adults. A larger problem is that efforts to limit the availability of drugs will tend to concentrate drug markets (and in turn hard-core drug use) in those communities whose social structure is least resistant to them. While it is hard to quantify the damage imposed by drug markets on poor urban communities, it is clear that drug markets worsen many of the conditions that social policy aims to improve. Locking up large numbers of young minority males in some urban communities may also have sharply negative consequences for those communities, including lower marriage rates, fewer children growing up in two-parent families, and less stable community composition. The sociologist William Julius Wilson gives considerable stress to the role of crime and drug selling in preventing the recovery of the most deprived urban communities.[12]

These concerns point to what may be a larger tension between drug policy and social policy. As William Brownsberger has noted, drug prohibition has very uneven distributional effects.[13] Our current prohibition appears largely successful from the vantage point of middle-class communities. Use and abuse of cocaine and heroin are, according to available measures, uncommon among the middle class. Moreover, middle-class neighborhoods are by and large insulated from the black market side effects of drug prohibition. Open drug selling and violence among dealers are almost unheard of in most better-off areas, as are the arrest and imprisonment of residents on drug charges. In contrast, residents of poor, urban neighborhoods do not fare so well. They suffer much higher rates of cocaine and heroin abuse (by more than a factor of ten, according to some measures),[14] the lion's share of the crime and violence attributable to illegal drug markets, and most of the punishment meted out by the criminal justice system for drug crimes.

Of course, poor urban communities also suffer a disproportionate share of the social problems that are the focus of social policy. Thus the distributional impact of our drug policy is roughly the opposite of the distributional objectives of many social policy programs. One could argue that the middle-class majority that benefits from our current drug policy has an obligation to try to remedy the resulting burdens placed on inner-city communities. One could also argue that since, short of repealing prohibition, there is only so much that drug policy narrowly defined can do to mitigate its distributional impact, remedies for poor communities will have to come from social policy programs. In any case, the fact that there are profound conflicts between the stated objectives of drug policy and social policy programs makes a strong case that there is a pressing need for better coordination of these policy realms.

The Structure of Current Drug Policy

Despite what seem to be strong arguments for a closer linkage between drug and social policy, current drug policy pays little attention to social programs. The annual *National Drug Control Strategy* (NDCS) released by the Office of National Drug Control Policy (ONDCP) is the most widely disseminated articulation of drug policy in this country and serves as the target for most discussion. It is focused almost exclusively on programs that aim to directly reduce drug use—mostly the number who use (prevalence) but arguably the quantities as well[15]—through enforcement, treatment, and prevention. Programs designed to address social conditions that give rise to drug use, or drug programs designed with social policy considerations in mind, are not an explicit part of the national strategy.

Interestingly, the 1997 NDCS and the subsequent document intended to provide a performance assessment system for policy decisions[16] for the first time explicitly recognized that ONDCP must be concerned with adverse consequences. The third of the five NDCS goals is to "reduce the health and social costs of drug use." This would appear to be an obvious opening to various social programs, yet for that purpose the strategy lists only drug treatment in addition to programs that reduce prevalence. The implicit premise is that nothing can directly target harms.

Indeed, the standard categorization of programs into demand reduction and supply reduction makes this point clear: a program that reduces the adverse consequences of drug use is neither of those. Consider needle exchange. Even its proponents are willing to accept that needle exchange might not decrease drug use (quantity or prevalence), but they claim that it has a substantial impact on a major adverse consequence of illicit drug use, namely the spread of HIV. If the federal government were to fund needle-exchange programs, it would be impossible to classify them as demand or supply reduction. They are purely harm reduction, as is methadone maintenance if one defines the problem as opiate addiction rather than addiction to illegal drugs. The fact that needle exchange does not fit into the usual split probably contributes to its lack of political acceptability.

Yet the American drug problem is obviously much more than the consumption of illegal intoxicants. It also encompasses the specific harms that come from the sale, production, and purchase of those drugs. There are programs that reduce the violence around drug markets (by targeting police resources not on drug selling itself but on related violence); increase the speed with which heroin addicts get treatment for hepatitis C (by providing better health access to poor adult males); or limit the visibility of disordered and fear-arousing drug addicts on streets (through order maintenance patrol activities). These all offer to reduce the adverse consequences of illicit drugs and have a strong claim to be included in the domain of drug policy. That does not so far get them on the NDCS score sheet, however.

This focus on use is consistent with the annual federal drug-control budget, a document accompanying the NDCS that is scrutinized carefully for the balance between supply reduction and demand reduction. The treatment of a patient with congestive heart failure resulting from frequent and sustained use of cocaine or heroin will not appear as drug treatment. Such expenditures are, after all, only concerned with a consequence of drug use, not with the use itself.

The resulting omissions from the drug budget are quite striking. For example, the only National Institutes of Health (NIH) programs considered relevant to the drug problem are those of the National Institute on Drug Abuse (NIDA).[17] In 1998 NIDA spent about $150 million on AIDS research, a small share of the nearly $1 billion invested by NIH in research on the disease, for which at least one-third of the cases have intravenous drug use as a primary risk factor. But because these other expenditures occur in other settings, with broader target populations, they are not included in the drug budget.[18]

There are odd exceptions to this, instances in which the treatment of symptoms is taken as an element of drug control. For example, in 1997 the catalog of drug treatment expenditures included $118 million by the Department of Education. One hardly thinks of this as an agency that provides such services, and indeed it does not. The expenditures were primarily for vocational rehabilitation programs "that assist individuals with a drug-related disabling condition."[19] Perhaps that expenditure, by enhancing the clients' educational performance, reduces their substance abuse problems, but no such argument is presented for its inclusion. But once this expenditure is allowed as an element of drug control, then a whole range of social services become eligible and total drug-control expenditures become very large indeed. After all, public-sector health and social expenditures related to use of illicit drugs total $45 billion,[20] and direct control costs account for less than two-thirds of that.

The Safe and Drug Free Schools Act (SDFSA) points to a different type of ambiguity. Descended from the Drug Free Schools Act, which was supposedly devoted to drug prevention alone, SDFSA provides broad funding for activities ranging from paving a path to a basketball court (recreation as prevention) to metal detectors for schools to help keep guns out (safer school environment)—that is, funding for almost anything that could be linked to lowering crime or drug use in school settings or by schoolchildren. The SDFSA embodies a view that drug use is not an isolated behavior to be dealt with in separate stand-alone programs but is a delinquency linked to others and to the environment in which the child develops; presumably (though it is not demonstrated), safe schools provide settings in which kids are less likely to turn to drugs.

These programs are the exceptions, though. In general, drug policy is narrowly considered for budget purposes to be only those programs that explicitly aim to reduce the extent of drug use or the quantity consumed by current users. And so the budgetary framework leaves little room for considerations of social policy.

The NDCS also pays no attention to the opposing link, namely the effects of drug policy on social problems. That tough drug enforcement might have adverse consequences for communities or individuals is never mentioned. This probably reflects both the emphasis on prevalence as the principal measure of success for drug policy and the broader social reluctance to face up to these inconvenient consequences.

Drug Use and Public Assistance

In asking whether policymakers should try to better coordinate policy programs currently thought of as drug and social policy, we are asking whether the strategic objectives of these policy areas should be expanded.[21] Should drug policy, which is now focused almost exclusively on reducing drug use, give explicit consideration to how it might reinforce or undermine social policy efforts? Should social policy programs, mostly designed to provide social services and income support, also seek to reduce drug use?

As we have discussed, one reason to be cautious about answering yes to these questions is that budgetary decisions and institutional arrangements tend to conform to existing conceptions of policy areas. While this creates a significant impediment to rethinking policy goals, it is not always insurmountable. Perhaps a more serious concern is that agencies are poorly equipped to manage a more complicated set of objectives or a broader range of responsibilities.

There is at best a weak relationship between the intended and actual effects of drug policy programs, and not only because of the ancillary consequences (both positive and negative) noted earlier. The public, and perhaps most policymakers as well, appears to view drug enforcement as a crime control program and publicly funded drug treatment as more of a public health effort. Yet this view probably sees things backwards. As Mark Moore has noted, it is likely that the largest benefit of publicly funded treatment is reduced crime, while the chief value of enforcement, which may increase or reduce crime depending on the circumstances, is reduced drug consumption.[22] Moreover, the link between many drug policy efforts and their supposed outcomes is in practice less than clear. There is, after all, strikingly little evidence that increases in drug enforcement or prevention (as presently implemented) actually have an effect on drug use or drug harms.

To put this another way: despite a narrowly defined mission and relatively settled institutional arrangements and responsibilities, current drug policy is widely misunderstood, and its practical effects are empirically uncertain. It would not be surprising, then, if it was extremely difficult to effectively link the goals of drug and social policy programs. The expansion of missions could lead to normative and political conflicts among goals; agencies might have to carry out tasks for which they were not designed; and uncertainty about the effects of policy actions could be even greater than it is now.

The use of public assistance funds to support drug habits provides a case in point. According to ONDCP, Americans spend over $50 billion annually on illegal drugs.[23] To our knowledge, no one has attempted to calculate what public assistance—such as Temporary Assistance to Needy Families (TANF), Supplemental Security Income (SSI), and Food Stamps—contributes to this total, but the figure is probably substantial. As Kleiman and Brownsberger emphasize in their chapters, heavy drug users account for a substantial share of total drug consumption. And because these users typically spend a very high share of whatever disposable income they have on drugs, one can reasonably infer that any public assistance they receive is primarily being spent on drugs.

One of the best sources of data on male heavy drug users has been the National Institute of Justice's Drug Use Forecasting program (DUF)—recently expanded and renamed the Arrestee Drug Abuse Monitoring (ADAM)—which administers drug tests and interviews to a sample of arrestees in major cities. According to DUF interviews, drug-using arrestees as a group obtain approximately 20 percent of their drug money from public assistance, principally SSI.[24] Female drug abusers are more likely to obtain drug money from various forms of welfare support, which together are much more generous than SSI. Treatment programs report that a large share of female participants are welfare recipients, although exact figures are not available.[25] All in all, it is not implausible that public assistance supports something between $5 and $10 billion in illicit drug spending, assuming that ONDCP's estimate of total spending is in the ballpark.

For many, this figure will spark outrage. But even those who accept it as the consequence of even a modest concern with poverty in a wealthy society must at least wonder if behavioral requirements for eligibility for public assistance can be used to address drug use in the recipient population. Two classes of requirement merit consideration: (1) an otherwise universal benefit is made contingent on the recipient being drug-free; and (2) drug impairment is one basis for eligibility in a particularistic program. We focus on income support programs because they have been the principal battlefront, though abstinence could be used more generally as a condition for any kind of public benefit, such as public housing tenancy or enrollment in job training programs.

Universal Programs

Consider the requirement that recipients of public assistance (in particular TANF) demonstrate abstinence from illicit drugs. At least eight states have declared their intention to test recipients for recent drug use and make continued abstinence a condition for continued receipt of TANF.[26] Those who test positive would be required to enter a treatment program or find some alternative means of abstaining. Failure to desist would be grounds for termination.

The justification here is principally, though not exclusively, reducing drug use in a population that is reputed to have high drug involvement, though as noted earlier that claim is disputed by some recent analyses.[27] Other justifications are possible. For example, those who use drugs are at greater risk of being abusive parents; adult TANF recipients are eligible because they are parents of dependent children. Though it is probable that drug use (as opposed to drug dependence or abuse) accounts for a small share of child abuse and neglect in this population, the relative simplicity of drug testing and the difficulty of assessing the other risk conditions give this justification some plausibility.

Preliminary inquiries suggest that no state had managed to implement the testing requirement as of early 1999, two and a half years after enactment of TANF. Consider for example the state of Maryland, which required under the new law that all TANF applicants have a Medicaid health examination within 30 days of registering for the program; the examination should include a screen for substance abuse. In fact the health providers screen using only a written set of questions, which, in the context of eligibility determination, are known to produce substantial underreporting. Urinalysis has not been used. As a consequence only about 100 applicants have been classified as in need of drug treatment so far, an implausibly low number given the thousands screened each year. In other states a pencil-and-paper test is administered as part of the application process in the human services office, with similarly few drug users being detected.

The reasons for failure to implement serious drug testing are no doubt many, from the logistic difficulty of implementing testing in welfare offices, which are required to make this determination in many states, to the cost of testing. But the lack of any directive that these human services agencies be concerned about drug use, except as it affects employability, reinforces the agency reluctance to take this responsibility seriously.

TANF may represent an important missed opportunity because it allows for the offer of positive incentives for abstinence. Payment of the next week's benefits could be dependent on a clean test for those who initially failed drug testing; after some period of negative tests, the recipient would move to less frequent testing and then to none.

A problem is that drug testing is a blunt instrument. A large fraction of positive tests are likely to be for occasional marijuana use.

Though such use is not without adverse consequences, it is difficult to make a strong case for being so intrusive in recipients' lives for such a modest gain in social functioning. Restricting the tests to drugs with much clearer harms, particularly cocaine, heroin, and methamphetamines, would make the case for testing more powerful and the rewards in terms of reduced drug-related harms more substantial.

The use of coercion to obtain abstinence among program recipients can also be justified by the potentially exacerbating effect of cash transfers on drug abuse. Public assistance, especially when given in cash or easily marketable vouchers such as food stamps, can provide resources for drug purchases. It is by now well documented that increases in public assistance to addicts result in increased drug consumption. For example, Andrew Shaner and his colleagues at the West Los Angeles Veterans Affairs Medical Center found that cocaine use among schizophrenics being treated on an outpatient basis was much higher at the beginning of the month, when many of the patients received their benefit checks.[28] The relationship seems to have both economic and psychological explanations. Because destitute addicts, who constitute a substantial proportion of those dependent on cocaine and heroin, have no savings (economists would say they are "liquidity constrained"), income is immediately spent on whatever increases self-perceived utility, which for addicts includes drugs. And this behavioral mechanism is then reinforced by another: cash becomes a conditioned cue for drug use. Note as well that, by making drug habits more manageable, public assistance reduces an addict's incentive to enter treatment.

Testing might in theory even have a broader deterrent effect. If a consequence of becoming drug dependent is the inability to meet eligibility requirements for TANF when one needs it, then some persons might not experiment with drugs earlier, knowing that experimentation runs the risk of dependence. This requires assumptions about foresight before the age of 20 (the age by which almost all drug users have initiated) that make it implausible. It is nonetheless the rationale that seems to underlie one component of TANF, the so-called Gramm Amendment. Anyone convicted of a drug felony after August 22, 1996 (the date of enactment) is denied TANF or Food Stamps benefits for life. It is difficult to explain why drug felonies should be singled out from all other felonies, unless it is for the deterrent effect on drug use itself.

The SSI program, a means-tested program created in 1972 that provides income for persons who are needy and aged, blind, or disabled, offers a useful middle-ground case. Like TANF, it is an income support program in which individual benefits are unrelated to any prior payments. However, eligibility is based on some fundamental characteristic (age, disability) that is covered by the social contract; in a liberal democracy the aged or disabled are assumed not to be able to support themselves through work. That SSI discourages workforce participation by some recipients is regrettable but not relevant here; all such benefits have disincentive effects.[29]

Targeted Programs

But if cash payments may exacerbate drug use, what are we to make of programs that provide support for those whose problems are very explicitly the consequence of drug dependence? Such programs are exemplified by the former SSI Drug Addiction and/or Alcoholism (DA&A) program, under which those whose long-term dependence on illicit drugs (or alcohol) induced such damage as to render them incapable of holding a job were eligible for a monthly government stipend in perpetuity. Eligibility rested not on dependence itself but on the consequences of that dependence; typically SSI eligibility was achieved only many years after the onset of drug dependence.

In December 1992, 5.2 million persons (about 2 percent of the total population) were receiving federal SSI payments averaging $330 per month.[30] SSI constitutes a major transfer program and contributes substantially to poverty alleviation in this country. From SSI's inception in 1972, a diagnosis of DA&A was included as a disability, along with various physical and mental handicaps, though large numbers of those who were drug dependent received benefits because of other disabilities consequent on long-term addiction, including organic brain disease and psychiatric co-morbidities.

However, DA&A recipients were uniquely singled out from other recipients of SSI. "The objective of the SSI DA&A program is to rehabilitate addicts to be productive members of society and remove them from the SSI disability rolls."[31] Hence those receiving SSI because of alcoholism or drug dependence were, in principle, required to be in treatment for that dependence; they were also required to have a custodian ("representative payee") who received their benefits. Other disability groups, including those with psychiatric problems, were subject to less stringent payment and treatment requirements.

In 1983, 10 years after its creation, the enrollment in DA&A was minuscule, only 3,000 persons. Then two states, California and Illinois, discovered that they could shift significant numbers of state welfare recipients onto the federal rolls. Enrollment rose to 20,000 recipients in 1990 and then 80,000 in 1994.[32] Without a change in rules it was estimated that the figure would rise to over 200,000 by the year 2000. If one included those with DA&A as a secondary diagnosis, the figure for 1994 was 250,000.

Few of those receiving SSI DA&A funds were in fact in treatment; most of the custodians were family members who probably made little effort to monitor the use of the income. A government study found that of those enrolled in June 1990, 70 percent were still receiving DA&A payments in February 1994; another 6 percent of those enrollees were receiving SSI payments under some other disability classification. Of the remainder, half (12 percent of the total) were deceased. Only 1 percent left the SSI rolls because of significant improvement in their earnings or medical status.[33] Clearly the program was not meeting the goal of helping addicts in their transition to sobriety and self-support.

The media reported horror stories of government checks being turned over to the local bar owner or drug dealer for purchase of alcohol or drugs.[34] The problem was exacerbated by the fact that, in the interests of fairness and recognizing the innate slowness of the bureaucratic process, SSI applicants received an initial lump-sum payment covering the months from first filing of a claim to time of enrollment. This could amount to $5,000 or more, and these initial payments generated the most egregious incidents.

The DA&A law itself had two glaring loopholes that undermined its potential effectiveness. First, treatment was required only when "available," and the DA&A enrollees could select their own representative payees. Second, the law created a disincentive for succeeding in treatment, since if a DA&A recipient overcame his addiction he would no longer be eligible for benefits. Nor was the Social Security Administration well equipped for the task of enforcing treatment. It is a check-writing agency, skilled in determination of eligibility but unpracticed at measuring compliance with a complex behavioral requirement such as participation in drug treatment. Eventually, it was frustration over the failure to get DA&As into treatment, combined with a view that drug users were undeserving of disability assistance, that led Congress to effectively eliminate the DA&A line of SSI.

Not surprisingly, the program came under strong attack in Congress. As a Congressional Research Service analysis concluded: "[The program] results in a perverse incentive that affronts working taxpayers and fails to serve the interests of addicts and alcoholics."[35] The SSI rules were first changed so that DA&A recipients had to leave the SSI rolls within three years; the representative payee and treatment enrollment requirements were to be rigorously enforced. Then in 1996 Congress decided that this basis for SSI eligibility was inappropriate and abolished the DA&A program.

Ironically, most of those forced off the DA&A rolls will probably find their way back to the SSI rolls for some other disability, in which even the minimal effort to prevent misuse of their government supports (requiring participation in treatment, use of responsible payees) will be missing. Long-term frequent use of cocaine and heroin often leads to increasing psychiatric problems that are disabling and thus lead to eligibility under other SSI provisions.

Could the DA&A program have accomplished much if it had enforced its payee and treatment provisions effectively? It is hard to reach a firm conclusion. Treatment drop-out rates are notoriously high for long-term drug users; retaining 50 percent of clients for 12 months is unusual.[36] It is true that clients do not generally lack for negative incentives, including avoidance of prison, but possibly the offer of money as a reward for abstinence would provide a powerful addition. The DA&A program would have no doubt helped some addicts, but there is not a strong basis for believing that it would have dramatically increased treatment retention rates among recipients. The notion of DA&A as a scholarship for treatment, without much more aggressive testing, was naïve.

Moreover, those who have been addicted to cocaine or heroin for a decade or more are at high risk of being unable to support themselves. A large literature shows that most of those dependent on drugs such as cocaine and heroin have a lifetime, chronic, relapsing condition.[37] Even those treatment subjects who greatly reduce their drug use do not do well in the labor market; for example, Hser, Anglin, and Powers found that 32 percent of the inactive users in their 24-year longitudinal study were unemployed at the time of the most recent interview.[38] Most evaluations find that it is reductions in crime that generate most of the economic benefits of treatment, not increased earnings.[39] Success in treatment would move them from the "poor addict" category to the "poor recovering addict" category, still requiring government support. Society will have to provide for them through some mechanism; the question is whether it is useful or appropriate to make their drug dependence explicitly the basis for that support.

Even if cash assistance makes addicts worse off, society still might choose to provide it. One reason is that cash assistance may reduce income-generating crime among addicts. The logic is straightforward labor economics. Addicts desire both leisure and drugs; public assistance allows them to obtain more of both. This appears to be at least a partial explanation of why heroin addicts in New York consume less heroin and commit more crime and do more legitimate work than their counterparts in Amsterdam, where social welfare payments are more generous.[40]

The poor (even the undeserving) have a call on a liberal democracy's largesse. Moreover, public assistance to addicts may reduce their criminal activity and thus improve the welfare of other citizens. Giving cash to poor addicts cannot be the ideal approach to alleviating their poverty. But ideal is not the same as realistic, and if paternalistic arrangements—such as enforced treatment with cash assistance paid to a trustee—are not feasible, then direct cash assistance, while not in the *best* interests of addicts, may be better both for the addict and for society than the alternative of no assistance.

But our purpose is not come to a judgment about whether addicts should be eligible for support either in universal programs or through targeted efforts. It is simply to suggest that this is a major issue for those interested in drug problems and the welfare of drug users. Yet it is not considered a part of the drug policy agenda; instead it is left to social policy discussions in which drug issues are at best second order.

Political Considerations

In both academic theory and government practice, public policy tends to be divided according to subject areas. There is defense policy and a Defense Department; international affairs and a State Department; transportation policy and a Transportation Department. There are both benefits and costs to drawing such lines. Making distinctions among policy subjects facilitates specialization, allowing individuals and organizations to develop expertise; it enhances efficiency through division of labor and organization of public management. On the downside, the distinctions are somewhat artificial—policy issues always cross subject boundaries (hence the vast number of interagency taskforces)—and they often make it difficult to identify and capitalize on opportunities for policy improvement that would require thinking or working across policy subjects.

As we have seen, analysis of both drug policy and social policy can be improved, at least at a high level of abstraction, by considering their effects on each other. In principle, it would seem that drug policy would be more beneficial if decisionmakers paid more attention to the negative social consequences of its actions, while social policy could help if it addressed drug addiction in its programs. Alas, there are institutional complications on both sides.

ONDCP was created for many reasons, ranging from the desire of a Democratic Congress to have a single Republican official to interrogate when the drug war was going badly, to a belief that the drug problem was so distinct and important that it needed a high-level official with no other responsibilities and substantial resources. The latter belief spawned efforts to create similar offices at the state and local levels. The Kennedy School of Government at Harvard even held training sessions for state and local drug czars in the early 1990s, yet by the late 1990s these offices had all but disappeared. As with the creation of ONDCP, many factors played a role. A new office, whose principal responsibility is coordination across other agencies and which has little budget authority, will not lack for strong bureaucratic enemies. In addition, these new institutions were less politically attractive to governors and legislatures when the drug problem moved from the headlines to just another item on the list of inner-city ills.

But we think that there may have been more substantive reasons than jealousy for the failure of these institutions. The policy levers that affect drug use and related problems are embedded in numerous programs, even within the criminal justice system. At neither the state nor the local level is there the array of specialized institutions dealing almost exclusively with drug problems (such as the Drug Enforcement Administration, NIDA, and the Substance Abuse and Mental Health Services Administration) that one finds at the federal level. Even police, though they have drug units, distribute their activities against dealers and users across a whole range of general units, from patrol through homicide investigation. The most important drug decisions within the police department may be those about criteria for allocation of effort by nonspecialized units. Should locations with open drug markets receive more patrol activity than would otherwise be warranted by the volume of complaints? How aggressively should homicide investigators pursue drug-related murders relative to others? These decisions are not transparent to any outside official. They can only be affected if the police management develops benchmarks that allow it to track how well the department deals with drug problems.[41]

Sadly, the history of efforts to link drug policy with other policy areas even at the federal level is not encouraging. Analysis of how the Department of Veterans Affairs (VA) is controlled politically points to the difficulties of a drug policy that tries to focus just on those programs that are explicitly concerned with controlling illicit drugs. The VA accounts for 40 percent of the federal treatment budget; its $1.1 billion budget is actually larger than that of the Substance Abuse and Mental Health Services Administration ($950 million), the dominant focus of tussles about treatment funding. The VA's decisions about what services to offer in its hospitals and how aggressively to disseminate information about them can have a major influence on treatment access for the drug dependent generally, given the prevalence of drug problems among veterans from the Vietnam era. However, these decisions are buried within a large, multi-service health services agency;

there is no single locus of budgetary decisionmaking for Congress or ONDCP to target so as to influence the drug budget of the agency. The result is that ONDCP has apparently done little to challenge the VA's allocations; in effect it is treated as a social service agency that happens to reduce drug consumption.

The various political forces that prevented SSI from successfully providing public assistance and drug treatment to poor substance abusers make us reluctant to endorse what might otherwise seem like sensible efforts to coordinate drug policy and social policy. Ideally, drug tests of welfare clients reveal valuable information that would allow public authorities to provide mothers with appropriate drug treatment services. But one does not have to be a cynic to imagine how drug testing of welfare mothers could undermine the social-welfare elements of TANF. It might deter some women from seeking services because of fear of the consequences of revealing to authorities their drug-using habits, while others who prefer the cheaper high of an occasional marijuana cigarette to the hangovers and intoxication of alcohol would be angry at the selective policies of the agencies.

There are many potential lessons from the SSI DA&A experience. One that we draw is the difficulty of providing services to drug abusers when the client population is specifically identified in that way. Most of those who were dropped from SSI when DA&A was ended in 1996 were able to stay on the SSI rolls because of some other disability, either a psychiatric co-morbidity or a physical disability developed in the course of a long addiction career. Protected by the broader eligibility, they will actually be subject to less scrutiny and restriction than they were under the DA&A program. Whether they and society are better off as a result is debatable but almost certainly will not be debated precisely because they are no longer visibly the responsibility of drug policy.

Conclusion

Given the present state of drug policy politics, it is difficult to be hopeful about forging effective links between drug policy and social policy. Social policy makers may wish that drug policy makers tried to mitigate the negative effects of drug enforcement on poor urban communities and did more to prevent and treat drug abuse among disadvantaged populations. But in today's political climate, acknowledging the negative side effects of drug enforcement is seen as inconsistent with a tough stance on drugs, and drug policy makers are judged more than anything on trends in the National Household Survey on Drug Abuse, which is not much influenced by drug abuse in the poorest areas. So it is unlikely that the social policy makers will push for their desired changes in drug policy, or that they would be successful even if they did.

What is more likely is that politicians will make new demands of social policy by requiring abstinence or treatment on the part of recipients, for such demands generally meet with strong public approval. Bear in mind, though, what several chapters in this book have emphasized: quitting drugs usually involves several cycles of relapse and is best encouraged through a carefully balanced combination of carrots and sticks. To date, there is no evidence that social service agencies have the skills or political support to carry out such efforts in a way that actually benefits recipients, although we hope that the increasing role of state governments in social service provision will generate some effective models.

We also hope that drug policy makers will pay more attention to other programs in which drug use is not central. A drug czar who encourages federally funded job training programs to include help for their adolescent participants to deal with drug use or its consequences, or who encourages Enterprise Zones to select neighborhoods affected by drug markets, or who encourages public housing programs to consider the importance of design to hinder the formation of such markets, may do a great deal to reduce America's drug problem even without affecting the budget for drug control.

Notes

Jonathan Caulkins and Philip Heymann provided very helpful comments on drafts of this chapter.

1. Prevention is sometimes bundled together with treatment into a "demand reduction vs. supply reduction" debate, but the politically sensitive issue

has been treatment. Everyone is in favor of prevention, if only we knew how to do it. See John G. Haaga and Peter H. Reuter, "Prevention: The (Lauded) Orphan of Drug Policy," in Robert H. Coombs and Douglas Ziedonis, eds., *Handbook on Drug Abuse Prevention* (Boston: Allyn and Bacon, 1995), 3–17.

2. David F. Musto, *The American Disease: Origins of Narcotic Control*, 3rd ed. (New York: Oxford University Press, 1999).

3. National Institute of Justice, *1998 Annual Report on Drug Use among Adult and Juvenile Arrestees* (Washington, 1999).

4. David Boyum and Mark A. R. Kleiman, "Alcohol and Other Drugs," in James Q. Wilson and Joan Petersilia, eds., *Crime* (San Francisco: ICS Press, 1995), 295–326.

5. Hendrick J. Harwood, Douglas Fountain, and Gina Livermore, in *The Economic Costs of Alcohol and Drug Abuse in the United States, 1992* (Rockville, Md.: National Institute on Drug Abuse, Office of Science Policy and Communications, 1998), estimate that abuse of illicit drugs accounted for $5.5 billion in health expenditures in 1992, not including drug treatment.

6. For example, in many methadone maintenance programs patients hardly ever see a counselor, let alone a physician. See Richard A. Rettig and Adam Yarmolinsky, eds., *Federal Regulation of Methadone Treatment* (Washington: National Academy Press, 1995).

7. Christopher Jencks, *The Homeless* (Cambridge, Mass.: Harvard University Press, 1994). General Accounting Office, *Parental Substance Abuse: Implications for Children, the Child Welfare System, and Foster Care Outcomes*, GAO/T-HEHS-98–40 (Washington, 1997). Mark J. Chaffin, Kelly J. Kelleher, and Janice A. Hollenberg, "Onset of Physical Abuse and Neglect: Psychiatric, Substance Abuse, and Social Risk Factors from Prospective Community Data," *Child Abuse and Neglect* 20, no. 3 (1996): 191–203.

8. See Statement of Peter Reuter, House Subcommittee on Human Resources of the Committee on Ways and Means, *Protecting Children from the Impacts of Substance Abuse on Families Receiving Welfare*, 105th Cong., 1st sess., Oct. 28, 1997, 21–25. This does not mean that drug abuse accounts for a large fraction of welfare claims. Indeed, some researchers conducting preliminary analyses of the Temporary Assistance to Needy Families (TANF) population suggest that the share of welfare recipients now impaired by illicit drugs may be substantially below 10 percent.

9. Often little is known about how well a specific program, such as Head Start, affects its principal outcome target (educational attainment) or how much a change in that outcome will reduce drug problems.

10. See, e.g., Elliot Currie, *Reckoning: Drugs, the Cities and the American Future* (New York: Hill and Wang, 1993).

11. James E. Rosenbaum, "Black Pioneers: Do Their Moves to the Suburbs Increase Economic Opportunity for Mothers and Children?" *Housing Policy Debate* 2, no. 4 (1991), 1179–1214.

12. William Julius Wilson, *When Work Disappears: The World of the New Urban Poor* (New York: Random House, 1997).

13. William N. Brownsberger, "Prevalence of Frequent Cocaine Use in Urban Poverty Areas," *Contemporary Drug Problems* 24 (1997): 349–371.

14. A number of statistical series show this; each is imperfect but they cumulatively show a picture that is highly credible. For example, 71 percent of treatment admissions for crack smoking are among African Americans and the majority of those are in large center cities in which African Americans are mostly poor. See *Preliminary Estimates from the National Client Data System* (Rockville, Md.: Substance Abuse and Mental Health Services Administration, 1992). Similar conclusions can be drawn from statistics from the criminal justice and health care systems.

15. Drug treatment produces abstinence in a very small fraction of patients, but it does substantially reduce the quantity consumed. See C. Peter Rydell and Susan S. Everingham, *Controlling Cocaine: Supply versus Demand Control Programs* (Santa Monica: Rand, 1994). On the overemphasis on prevalence see Jonathan P. Caulkins and Peter Reuter, "Setting Goals for Drug Policy: Harm Reduction or Use Reduction?" *Addiction* 97, no. 9 (1997): 1143–50.

16. *Blueprint for a Drug Free America* (Washington: ONDCP, 1997).

17. A small amount of National Institute on Alcoholism and Alcohol Abuse spending, related to underage drinking, is also included because ONDCP's mandate covers use of alcohol by those under the legal drinking age of 21.

18. The Health Care Finance Administration (HCFA) and the Department of Veterans Affairs (VA), in describing their drug control budgets, show the inconsistencies that arise from this approach. HCFA states: "Only direct treatment costs have been estimated, to the exclusion of costs associated with the treatment of drug-related conditions." *National Drug Control Strategy, 1998: Budget Summary* (Washington: Office of National Drug Control Policy), 50. The VA states: "'Treatment Costs' represent the cost for all inpatient and outpatient care of veterans with a primary or associated diagnosis of drug abuse. These figures include the cost of care for these patients in the following: specialized drug abuse treatment programs; specialized substance abuse programs treating veterans with alcohol and/or drug abuse problems; and, all other medical programs (e.g., medicine, surgery, psychiatry, etc.)." Ibid., 204.

19. Ibid., 37.

20. Harwood, Fountain, and Livermore, *Economic Costs,* 1–7.

21. We are still defining policy areas in terms of *intent*. In this we differ from a much-cited study of crime prevention that defined its domain purely by *effect*: Lawrence W. Sherman, Denise Gottfredson, Doris MacKenzie, John Eck, Peter Reuter, and Shawn Bushway, "Preventing Crime: What Works, What Doesn't, What's Promising," Report to the U.S. Congress, Prepared for the National Institute of Justice (College Park: Department of Criminology and Criminal Justice, University of Maryland, 1997). Sherman and his colleagues wished to make the politically important point that crime prevention was indeed an effect and that many *programs* that prevent crime (e.g., home visits by nurses to families with young children) have other primary labels. We are more interested in policy than in programs.

22. Mark H. Moore, "Drugs, the Criminal Law, and the Administration of Justice," *Milbank Quarterly* 69, no. 4 (1991): 529–560.

23. William Rhodes, Stacia Langenbahn, Ryan Kling, and Paul Scheiman, *What America's Users Spend on Illegal Drugs, 1988–1995* (Washington: ONDCP, 1997).

24. David Boyum, "The DUF Cocaine/Crack and Heroin Addendum: Data and Information for Drug Policy," presented at the annual meeting of the American Society of Criminology, Chicago, Nov. 1996.

25. In some cities as many as one-third of 1997 ADAM female respondents reported welfare and Social Security as their principal sources of income in the previous 30 days. One study reports that 41 percent of California's female drug treatment clients in 1992 were in receipt of some public assistance, which could include General Assistance as well as AFDC. Dean R. Gerstein, Robert A. Johnson, Cindy L. Larison, Henrick J. Harwood, and Douglas Fountain, *Alcohol and Other Drug Treatment for Parents and Welfare Recipients: Outcomes, Costs, and Benefits* (Washington: U.S. Department of Health and Human Services, Office of the Assistant Secretary for Planning and Evaluation, 1997).

26. Legal Action Center, *Welfare Reform and Substance Abuse* (Washington, 1997). The federal legislation creating TANF (The Personal Responsibility and Work Opportunity Reconciliation Act) does not specify how the states should deal with substance abuse among clients; the primary incentive for the states to do so comes from the need to achieve high employment rates among welfare clients. The statute does allow for testing without requiring prior federal approval.

27. Bridget F. Grant and Deborah A. Dawson, "Alcohol and Drug Use, Abuse, and Dependence among Welfare Recipients," *American Journal of Public Health* 86, no. 10 (1996): 1450–54.

28. Andrew Shaner, Thad A. Eckman, Lisa J. Roberts, Jeffery N. Wilkins, Douglas E. Tucker, John W. Tsuang, and Jim Mintz, "Disability Income, Cocaine Use, and Repeated Hospitalization among Schizophrenic Co-

caine Abusers: A Government-Sponsored Revolving Door?" *New England Journal of Medicine* 333, no. 12 (1995): 777–783.

29. For many who are disabled, the decision to seek work is a function of incentives. Thus disability claims tend to fall as labor markets tighten. Deborah A. Stone, *The Disabled State* (Philadelphia: Temple University Press, 1984).

30. "Section IV: Income Support Programs," *Social Security Bulletin* 56, no. 4 (1993): 64–84.

31. General Accounting Office, *Social Security: Major Changes Needed for Disability Benefits for Addicts*, GAO/HEHS-94–128 (Washington, 1994), 4.

32. Department of Health and Human Services, Office of the Inspector General, *SSI Payments to Drug Addicts and Alcoholics: Continued Dependence*, OEI-09–94–007 (Washington, 1994).

33. Ibid.

34. See Christopher M. Wright, "SSI: The Black Hole of the Welfare State," *Policy Analysis*, no. 224 (Washington: Cato Institute, April 27, 1995).

35. Carmen Solomon, *Supplemental Security Income (SSI) Drug Addicts and Alcoholics: Welfare Reform in the 104th Congress* (Washington: Congressional Research Service, 1995).

36. Dean R. Gerstein and Hendrick J. Harwood, eds., *Treating Drug Problems,* vol. 1 (Washington: National Academy Press, 1990).

37. See M. Douglas Anglin and Yih-Ing Hser, "Treatment of Drug Abuse," in Michael Tonry and James Q. Wilson, eds., *Drugs and Crime* (Chicago: University of Chicago Press, 1990), 393–460.

38. Yih-Ing Hser, M. Douglas Anglin, and Keiko Powers, "A 24-Year Follow-Up of California Narcotics Addicts," *Archives of General Psychiatry* 50 (1993), 577–584.

39. See, e.g., Dean R. Gerstein, Robert A. Johnson, Hendrick J. Harwood, Douglas Fountain, Natalie Suter, and Kathryn Malloy, "Evaluating Recovery Services: The California Drug and Alcohol Treatment Assessment (CALDATA)," publication no. ADP 94–629 (Sacramento: California Department of Alcohol and Drug Programs, 1994).

40. Martin Grapendaal, Ed Leuw, and Hans Nelen, "Drugs and Crime in an Accommodating Social Context: The Situation in Amsterdam," *Contemporary Drug Problems* 19, no. 2 (1992): 303–326. Studies of addicts in Oslo and in Australian cities also provide some support for this; broad but shallow benefits moderate criminal involvement. See Anne Line Bretteville-Jensen and Matthew Sutton, "The Income Generating Behavior of Injecting Drug Users in Oslo," *Addiction* 91 (1996): 63–80; Wendy Loxley, Susan Carruthers, and Jude Bevan, *In the Same Vein: First Report of the Australian Study of HIV and Injecting Drug Use* (Perth: Australian National Center for Research into Prevention of Drug Abuse, 1995).

Needle and Mills found a much higher percentage of New York addicts in receipt of government transfers than did Johnson et al. ten years earlier, probably reflecting improved access to SSI and the aging of the addict population; they were also less criminally active. See Richard Needle and Arnold Mills, *Drug Procurement Practices of the Out-of-Treatment Chronic Drug Abuser* (Rockville, Md.: National Institute on Drug Abuse, 1994); Bruce D. Johnson, Paul J. Goldstein, Edward Preble, James Schmeidler, Douglas S. Lipton, Barry Spunt, and Thomas Miller, *Taking Care of Business: The Economics of Crime by Heroin Abusers* (Lexington, Mass.: Lexington Books, 1985).

41. The political autonomy of the local prosecutor (who is elected at the county level in most states) also creates problems for state or local drug czars.

Postscript

Philip B. Heymann

In the final analysis the two most important unanswered questions in U.S. policy toward cocaine and heroin are these. First, would it be wise to shift our commitment to using law enforcement to reduce the availability of these drugs back to something like the level of the Reagan years? Second, should we reconsider the way we are conducting a war on drugs to avoid thoughtlessly nourishing the conviction among minority groups that the United States does not accord them equal protection of the laws? The political and policy plausibility of making changes in response to these questions makes them far more urgent than the more familiar debate about some form of broad legalization, a proposal whose consequences would be likely to expand the use of these drugs far more than most Americans would now find acceptable.[1]

A second characteristic also makes these questions deserving of immediate attention. Getting the facts required for widely convincing answers—and there are highly relevant facts about which there can be real doubt—is critical, but it will take time. Our very inability to answer convincingly now has obvious implications for policy. As Sherlock Holmes remarked to Watson, the strongest evidence as to who had committed a certain crime was that the dog had not barked in the night. There are surprisingly strong conclusions for drug policy to be drawn from the absence of evidence—from our inability to answer these two questions conclusively.

265

Focus first on what we do not know about the effect of law enforcement on drug use: whether an increase or decrease of 25 percent or more in our expenditures on law enforcement would have any significant effect on limiting drug consumption. What we do know is discouraging, although far from conclusive. Massive increases in law enforcement in the last two decades did not prevent a substantial reduction in the price of a pure gram of heroin or cocaine. No one believes that the increased expenditures on law enforcement made drugs cheaper; there are a number of plausible explanations of why drugs became cheaper. But the fact remains that price went down and quality went up despite immense increases in law enforcement efforts.

Looking less globally at the issue of effectiveness of law enforcement is hardly more encouraging. Jonathan Caulkins has noted that there is no evidence that increases in high-level seizures in the United States are followed by price increases, and that many criminal statutes punish possession and sale of crack cocaine more severely than comparable powder cocaine offenses, but there are no systematic price differentials between cocaine in the form of crack and in the form of powder.[2] Nor does theory give hope; there are any number of reasons why devoting ever-increasing resources to the effort to raise the price or prevent the sale of illicit drugs might result in sharply reduced returns.[3]

While the experts may argue about the explanations for this evidence or, more realistically, the meaning of the absence of critical evidence, the question presented by Sherlock Holmes cries out for an answer: "What is the implication of the absence of evidence?" For this much is indisputably clear: we cannot detect any recent increase in price or reduction in trafficking despite having spent more and more money for law enforcement against drugs in recent years. While we cannot eliminate the possibility that at some level of increase of expenditure the rewards in terms of reduced drug use would suddenly become real or apparent, or that increased expenditures may have been useful as part of a valiant, rear-guard fight against other more powerful forces driving down the price of drugs and increasing their availability, we have no evidence now to support these possibilities. There is nothing that we could call more than guesses. Although legalizing drugs or cutting law enforcement by 95 percent would be likely to greatly increase use, there is no real evidence of what the effects of 25 percent more or less spent on law enforcement would be.

So let's return to Sherlock Holmes and look for the implications of silence. What do most people do when increasingly costly efforts are not producing any persuasive evidence of the desired results? The answers are familiar. Reduce the costly efforts and see if the results are as good without them. Try something new to reach the same desired results. Or, finally, use the costly resources to pursue other results. Each of these three would be far more sensible in the case of law enforcement against drugs than simply continuing to pour money and lives at the same or an increasing rate into an effort that provides no evidence of successful results from the last 25 percent in investment.

We should experiment with reducing the intensity and cost of law enforcement until we can detect an increase in drug use. We should look for alternative ways to spend law enforcement dollars to accomplish the same goals. Treatment and prevention are the major categories, but alternative forms of law enforcement, such as the controlled abstinence described by Mark Kleiman or other forms of testing, should also be pursued. We should look for uses of the last law enforcement dollars, perhaps not for agriculture or defense but for objectives that combine reduced drug use with other goals, such as reduced violence, protection of youth, reduced risk of diseases spread by dirty needles, increased neighborhood order and civility, and reduced disparities in enforcement.

There are, in short, intelligent ways to react to an absence of information or evidence as to whether the last 25 percent of the expenditures on a costly program of law enforcement is producing any significant incremental results. In the long run the most important reaction may be to take the steps necessary to produce the evidence. In the short run, experiment. Above all, suspect the normal human inclinations to try to justify past expenditures by "pouring good money after bad" or to "prove who's boss" in a contest of wills with those who ignore our prohibitions on certain use and sale of drugs. Our job is to reduce the costs of dependence and intoxication at the lowest cost in lives and dollars, not to prove that no one can defy law enforcement.

On the second great question we have some evidence, but it is conflicting. Very high percentages of our poor, urban, and minority populations believe both that drug use is a serious problem *and* that the

American war on drugs demonstrates that law enforcement is used unfairly against the population groups to which they belong. A *New York Times* survey in mid-2000 found that two-thirds of black Americans were convinced that the system of law enforcement was biased against them.[4] On the other hand, very high proportions of the white middle class believe that the problem presented by the sale and use of the most dangerous drugs, particularly cocaine and heroin, is concentrated in minority communities and that therefore expenditures on drug law enforcement not only are not discriminatory but are likely to benefit those communities most. The dispute creates a political division within the United States on an issue of law enforcement fairness and neutrality that is of immense importance to the social health of the nation.

What do we know about the fairness of the use of the two-thirds of expenditures on drug programs that go to law enforcement? We know from the two large surveys run by the federal government that there is no great disparity in the *reported* prevalence of use of drugs among blacks, whites, and Hispanics.[5] We have no good evidence on the percentage of dealers identified with a particular location, social or economic group, race, or ethnicity. We also know from figures from Massachusetts like those discussed by William Brownsberger and from equally astonishing figures from Illinois that there is often an immense disproportion in the percentage of each of these categories—particularly of racial and ethnic groups—that is sent to the penitentiary for drug crimes.[6] If the prevalence figures correspond even roughly to the proportions of individuals from different groups dealing drugs or the proportions who are heavy, addicted users—and the survey results are not adequate for reaching a conclusion on either of these matters—then something immensely unfair is at work in the operation of our criminal justice system, for the proportion of penitentiary sentences for blacks, Hispanics, and residents of certain urban areas is many times the average for whites.

Are the proportions of dealers and addicts from different population groups really as skewed as the penitentiary figures suggest? Or do the figures instead reflect a series of choices which have, intentionally or unintentionally, burdened one part of our population with the cost of law enforcement? Obviously, this issue is of central importance in terms of the overall credibility of the criminal justice system in the eyes of very large numbers of American citizens. The answer bears on what is and what is not wise drug policy in almost every area. It also affects the availability of community support for any of a variety of drug policy initiatives.

No responsible observer believes that one racial or ethnic group is innately more inclined to deal or use dangerous drugs than any other group. But *if* something in the social and economic structure leads to vastly more drug dealing (or drug addiction) by one group,[7] recognizing this frankly poses far less of a threat to a healthy American society than the belief that the largest part of our law enforcement efforts are deeply biased. On the other hand, if the cause of much of the disparity in prison sentences is not a great difference in the prevalence of dealing or addiction in different populations, then addressing the bias reflected in the vastly greater rates of imprisonment for minority groups is far more important than any loss in benefits from drug enforcement caused by addressing that bias. And the existence of bias is made more plausible by what historians of drug enforcement have taught us about the association in the public mind, 100 years ago, of opium use with Chinese immigrants, or 80 years ago of cocaine use with blacks, or of marijuana use with Mexicans in the 1930s.

Even if the likelihood of penitentiary sentences for dealing or abusing drugs is vastly excessive for one group in light of its overall involvement with illicit drugs, that may not mean that the group is an object of blatant discrimination. The difference in prison sentences may reflect differences in attitudes toward particular drugs or particular drug-related activity. Thus, who is sent to the penitentiary and who is not depends upon a variety of factors: what forms of drug use are criminalized; what the penalties are; what drugs and what situations of sale or use prosecutors believe are most dangerous; and enforcement against what drugs and in what situations is emphasized by the police. Disparities in treatment could result at any of these places and might not involve hostility to a racial or ethnic group. Still, the pattern of inequality would be very troublesome.

Consider some possibilities. Crack is a more dangerous drug than marijuana and, because of the way it is used, than powder cocaine. But its vastly more severe penalties under federal law may be attributable to the fact that the more powerful political constituencies are far more likely to know people who use marijuana or powder cocaine, and the least powerful minority constituencies are more likely to know people who use crack. Efforts to reduce the disparity between crack, a drug disproportionately used by blacks, and powder cocaine, the same drug in a nonsmokable form used by whites, may have failed for similar reasons. Prosecutors determine their priorities in large part by the applicable sentence, thereby picking up whatever prejudice goes into the definition of the crime and its sentence.

Investigators and police do the same, but are also influenced by the productivity in terms of arrests of particular forms of investigation. Outdoor drug dealing, far more common in poor neighborhoods, is also far easier to pursue than drug dealing in private in wealthier neighborhoods. If car "stops" justified by violations of traffic rules are used as a pretext to discover drugs, as the Supreme Court allows, the police are likely to choose drivers by whatever visible characteristics (race, class, and so on) even slightly increase the probability of finding drugs, although such "racial profiling" is likely to greatly distort the proportion of African Americans arrested compared to their proportion in the trafficking or using population.

In short, while some disparity in likelihood of prison sentences between two groups may be explained by differences in drug consumption and sales that really matter socially and morally, other explanations are almost as worrisome as blatant racism. Some involve displaying greater concern for one's constituents and friends than for other groups. Some unjustified disparities result from factual mistakes that no one bothers to correct—such as the misconception that crack dealers are drug kingpins—some from political calculation of the worst sort. But in the final analysis any governmental action—from setting the penalty for a particular drug to making arrests on the street—that creates great and indefensible disparities in prison sentences along racial or ethnic lines will undermine trust in the fairness of government and law enforcement. The health of American society, in a very fundamental way, depends upon our ability to justify to those who bear most of the cost of law enforcement any dramatic disparities in who is sent to prison.

In the long run, we must press for the needed facts and vigorously probe the justifications that lie behind the practices that lead to different groups bearing very different costs of law enforcement. But, until the facts are in, we should not risk encouraging deeply unsettling beliefs in governmental bias for any but the most compelling of reasons. For now we should take every step possible to eliminate disparities that we may well not be able to justify. An obvious starting point would be to end the peculiar system of mandatory minimum sentences for specific drugs, particularly the disparity between crack and powder cocaine, which the federal government has found to account for a very large part of the difference in likelihood of different groups being in federal penitentiaries. A next step would be to make continued availability of the power to "stop" on suspicion or the power to arrest and search on the pretext of a minor traffic violation contingent on a convincing showing that neither power is being used in a racially disparate manner.

Notes

1. The prices of cocaine and heroin would be a very small fraction of what they are now if the production of these drugs were legal. Radically reducing the price and totally removing the effect of legal prohibition in activating and reinforcing social condemnation of their use, let alone permitting the effects of advertising, would be extremely likely to result in sharply increased social acceptance of use, as in the case of alcohol.

2. Yuehong Yuan and Jonathan P. Caulkins, "The Effect of Variation in High-Level Domestic Drug Enforcement on Variation in Drug Prices," *Socio-Economic Planning Sciences* 32, no. 4 (1998); Jonathan P. Caulkins, "Is Crack Cheaper than (Powder) Cocaine?" *Addiction* 92, no. 11 (1997): 1437–43.

3. Later increments in expenditure would be expected to produce less than earlier ones, for the most profitable avenues for arrest of dealers or seizure of drugs would already have been exploited. Moreover, much of any increase in the price of the drugs would have to be traceable to higher salaries required to compensate for an increased risk of arrest with more law enforcement. But this assumes that those whose salaries represent the major cost of a drug-dealing operation would know the risk had increased.

4. *New York Times*, July 11, 2000.

5. The surveys do not reveal the number of very heavy users of any particular drug. Nor do they reveal the total amount of any drug used by any category of user. It is thus entirely possible that a relatively small percentage of

272   Drug Addiction and Drug Policy

total users *both* accounts for a high percentage of total use *and* is heavily concentrated in one population category. See M. E. Ensminger, J. C. Anthony, and J. McCord, "The Inner City and Drug Use," *Drug and Alcohol Dependence* 48 (1997): 175–184.

6. See M. Tonry, *Malign Neglect* (New York: Oxford University Press, 1995), ch. 3.

7. One obvious possibility regarding dealing involves the origin of certain drugs and established distribution patterns. The distribution system for all of our cocaine and much of our heroin starts in Colombia, works through Mexico and the Caribbean, and then on through the poverty areas of central cities, heavily populated by minorities.

Contributors

David Boyum, Ph.D. Vice President and Director of Policy Research and Analysis, BOTEC Analysis Corporation

William N. Brownsberger, J.D. Associate Director for Public Policy, Division on Addictions, Harvard Medical School

Jonathan Caulkins, Ph.D. Director of Pittsburgh Office, RAND Corporation

Gene M. Heyman, Ph.D. Harvard Medical School, McLean Hospital, North Charles Center on the Addictions

Philip B. Heymann, J.D. James Barr Ames Professor of Law, Harvard Law School

Mark A. R. Kleiman, Ph.D. Professor of Policy Studies, UCLA School of Public Policy

Mark H. Moore, Ph.D. Daniel and Florence Guggenheim Professor of Criminal Justice Policy and Management, John F. Kennedy School of Government, Harvard University

Peter Reuter, Ph.D. Professor, School of Public Affairs and Department of Criminology, University of Maryland

Sally L. Satel, M.D. Psychiatrist and Lecturer, Yale University

George E. Vaillant, M.D. Professor of Psychiatry, Harvard Medical School